Autoerotic Deaths

Practical Forensic and Investigative Perspectives

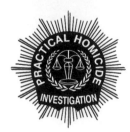

CRC SERIES IN
**PRACTICAL ASPECTS OF CRIMINAL
AND FORENSIC INVESTIGATIONS**

VERNON J. GEBERTH, BBA, MPS, FBINA *Series Editor*

**Practical Homicide Investigation: Tactics, Procedures, and
Forensic Techniques, Fourth Edition**
Vernon J. Geberth

**Practical Homicide Investigation Checklist and Field Guide,
Second Edition**
Vernon J. Geberth

Practical Military Ordnance Identification
Tom Gersbeck

Practical Cold Case Homicide Investigations Procedural Manual
Richard H. Walton

Autoerotic Deaths: Practical Forensic and Investigative Perspectives
Anny Sauvageau and Vernon J. Geberth

Practical Crime Scene Processing and Investigation, Second Edition
Ross M. Gardner

**The Counterterrorism Handbook: Tactics, Procedures, and Techniques,
Fourth Edition**
Frank Bolz, Jr., Kenneth J. Dudonis, and David P. Schulz

Practical Forensic Digital Imaging: Applications and Techniques
Patrick Jones

Practical Bomb Scene Investigation, Second Edition
James T. Thurman

Practical Crime Scene Investigations for Hot Zones
Jacqueline T. Fish, Robert N. Stout, and Edward Wallace

**Sex-Related Homicide and Death Investigation: Practical and Clinical
Perspectives, Second Edition**
Vernon J. Geberth

Handbook of Forensic Toxicology for Medical Examiners
D. K. Molina

Practical Crime Scene Analysis and Reconstruction
Ross M. Gardner and Tom Bevel

Serial Violence: Analysis of Modus Operandi and Signature Characteristics of Killers
Robert D. Keppel and William J. Birnes

Practical Aspects of Rape Investigation: A Multidisciplinary Approach, Fourth Edition
Robert R. Hazelwood and Ann Wolbert Burgess

Bloodstain Pattern Analysis: With an Introduction to Crime Scene Reconstruction, Third Edition
Tom Bevel and Ross M. Gardner

Tire Tread and Tire Track Evidence: Recovery and Forensic Examination
William J. Bodziak

Officer-Involved Shootings and Use of Force: Practical Investigative Techniques, Second Edition
David E. Hatch and Randy Dickson

Informants and Undercover Investigations: A Practical Guide to Law, Policy, and Procedure
Dennis G. Fitzgerald

Practical Drug Enforcement, Third Edition
Michael D. Lyman

Cold Case Homicides: Practical Investigative Techniques
Richard H. Walton

Practical Analysis and Reconstruction of Shooting Incidents
Edward E. Hueske

Principles of Bloodstain Pattern Analysis: Theory and Practice
Stuart James, Paul Kish, and T. Paulette Sutton

Global Drug Enforcement: Practical Investigative Techniques
Gregory D. Lee

Practical Investigation of Sex Crimes: A Strategic and Operational Approach
Thomas P. Carney

Principles of Kinesic Interview and Interrogation, Second Edition
Stan Walters

Practical Criminal Investigations in Correctional Facilities
William R. Bell

Practical Aspects of Interview and Interrogation, Second Edition
David E. Zulawski and Douglas E. Wicklander

Forensic Pathology, Second Edition
Dominick J. Di Maio and Vincent J. M. Di Maio

The Practical Methodology of Forensic Photography, Second Edition
David R. Redsicker

Quantitative-Qualitative Friction Ridge Analysis: An Introduction to Basic and Advanced Ridgeology
David R. Ashbaugh

Footwear Impression Evidence: Detection, Recovery, and Examination, Second Edition
William J. Bodziak

Gunshot Wounds: Practical Aspects of Firearms, Ballistics, Forensic Techniques, Second Edition
Vincent J. M. Di Maio

The Sexual Exploitation of Children: A Practical Guide to Assessment, Investigation, and Intervention, Second Edition
Seth L. Goldstein

Practical Aspects of Munchausen by Proxy and Munchausen Syndrome Investigation
Kathryn Artingstall

Practical Fire and Arson Investigation, Second Edition
David R. Redsicker and John J. O'Connor

Interpretation of Bloodstain Evidence at Crime Scenes, Second Edition
William G. Eckert and Stuart H. James

Investigating Computer Crime
Franklin Clark and Ken Diliberto

Practical Investigation Techniques
Kevin B. Kinnee

Friction Ridge Skin: Comparison and Identification of Fingerprints
James F. Cowger

Tire Imprint Evidence
Peter McDonald

Practical Gambling Investigation Techniques
Kevin B. Kinnee

Anny Sauvageau
Vernon J. Geberth

Autoerotic Deaths

Practical Forensic and Investigative Perspectives

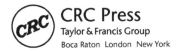

CRC Press
Taylor & Francis Group
Boca Raton London New York

CRC Press is an imprint of the
Taylor & Francis Group, an **informa** business

CRC Press
Taylor & Francis Group
6000 Broken Sound Parkway NW, Suite 300
Boca Raton, FL 33487-2742

First issued in paperback 2021

© 2013 by Taylor & Francis Group, LLC
CRC Press is an imprint of Taylor & Francis Group, an Informa business

No claim to original U.S. Government works

Version Date: 20130308

ISBN 13: 978-0-367-78117-0 (pbk)
ISBN 13: 978-1-4398-3712-2 (hbk)

Visit the Taylor & Francis Web site at
http://www.taylorandfrancis.com

and the CRC Press Web site at
http://www.crcpress.com

Contents

Preface

Autoerotic Deaths

Practical Forensic and Investigative Perspectives is the result of a meticulous collaboration and friendship between a former New York detective and homicide commander, who is now an international homicide and forensic consultant, and an experienced forensic pathologist, who is the chief medical examiner of Alberta and an internationally recognized authority on asphyxial death. This book is the result of a unique combination of the knowledge and experience of a dedicated murder cop who has seen it all and that of a passionate scientist whose research in the field has modernized the concepts around autoerotic deaths. The two authors have enjoyed multiple conversations during which the new data of the science met the concrete examples of case studies. This is what this book is all about: presenting a scientific modern view of autoerotic death, with case illustrations.

Autoerotic Deaths: Practical Forensic and Investigative Perspectives will become the benchmark and "best practice" model for professional death investigations involving autoerotic deaths because it will provide practical and conventional information based on scientific research and case experience from the field with a wide variety of exquisite case histories.

Throughout this textbook, we reference additional resource information as well as case examples of the application of various tactics, procedures, and forensic techniques along with full-color illustrations, explanations, and tables to assist the reader in understanding the dynamics of autoerotic deaths.

In Chapter 1, a historical context of the evolution of the concept of sexual asphyxia and autoerotic death is presented. The appearance and development of the phenomenon is followed from the early nonscientific reports in the French literature and the whorehouses of London, through the early scientific reports (1947 to 1980), the golden age of the wide development of the field mainly under the team of Hazelwood (1981 to 1990), to the turning point of a revolutionary paper by Byard and Bramwell (1991) and the modern era that followed.

In Chapter 2, the definition of autoerotic death is presented, along with the pitfalls in the application of the term *autoerotic*: (1) to label a death autoerotic even though the manner of death was not accidental, (2) to label a death autoerotic even though the sexual asphyxia was not solitary, and (3) to become confused concerning the concept of an escape mechanism. The incidence of autoerotic death is reviewed, and the best practices in approaching these deaths are discussed.

In Chapter 3, the death scene characteristics are explored. As the main clues to the autoerotic nature of a death are at the scene, this chapter is particularly important. The most common scene features are exposure of genitals, pornography, nudity, cross-dressing, and bondage.

The methods of autoerotic deaths are explored in Chapters 4–6. The most common method of autoerotic death is hanging (explored in Chapter 4), followed at some distance by asphyxia by plastic bags and chemical substances (Chapter 5). Unusual methods are presented in Chapter 6: electrocution, overdressing/body wrapping, foreign body insertion, and atypical asphyxia.

Finally, Chapter 7 discusses the atypical victims of autoerotic deaths: the female victims, the non-white victims, the teenager, and elderly victims.

We would like to particularly thank Mark Benecke, international forensic research and consulting, for his contribution to Chapters 4 and 5 and Brian Wilson, director of production, Medicolegal Art (Atlanta, GA) for his exquisite medical drawings and illustrations.

Autoerotic Deaths: Practical Forensic and Investigative Perspectives presents a complete analysis of all aspects of autoerotic deaths. Our goal was to develop a comprehensive resource text that could serve as a practical guide for those involved in the investigation of such deaths. We hope readers will appreciate the combination of theory and practice, with this unique combination of the most up-to-date science presented in parallel to a more practical, down-to-earth case history format.

Anny Sauvageau and Vernon J. Geberth

About the Authors

Anny Sauvageau, MD, MSc, Chief Medical Examiner, Alberta, Canada

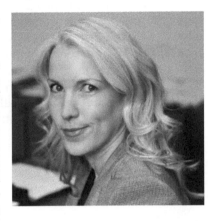

Dr. Anny Sauvageau started her career as a forensic pathologist in Montreal in 2002. In 2009, she moved to Alberta, Canada, where she was named deputy chief medical examiner in 2010 and chief medical examiner in 2011. She is an associate clinical professor at the University of Alberta and the University of Calgary and a well-known world expert on asphyxia. She received her medical degree from the University of Montreal in 1996 and was board certified in anatomical pathology in 2002. She has a founder designation in forensic pathology from the Royal College of Physicians and Surgeons of Canada in recognition of her significant contribution to the development of this new specialty in Canada. From 2007 to 2012, she was vice president of the Forensic Pathology Examination Board of the Royal College of Physicians and Surgeons of Canada. She is also one of the founders and the program director of the residency program in forensic pathology at the University of Alberta. She is the author of more than 75 papers in peer-reviewed forensic journals and a much sought-after international speaker. She is the founder of the Working Group on Human Asphyxia and the cofounder of the International Network for Forensic Research. Her innovative approach toward forensic research has significantly improved the understanding of the pathophysiology of hanging and other types of strangulation.

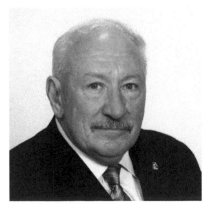

Vernon J. Geberth, MS, MPS, BBA, Lieutenant Commander (Ret.) NYPD, Practical Homicide Investigation® (http://www.practicalhomicide.com)

Commander Vernon Geberth is a retired lieutenant commander of the New York City Police Department with over 40 years of law enforcement experience. He has an undergraduate degree in business administration and holds dual master's degrees in forensic psychology and criminal justice. Commander Geberth is a graduate of the Federal Bureau of Investigation (FBI) National Academy and is also a Fellow in the American Academy of Forensic Sciences (AAFS).

Lieutenant Commander Geberth is the author of *Practical Homicide Investigation: Tactics, Procedures, and Forensic Techniques,* now in its fourth edition and recognized in the law enforcement field as "the bible of homicide investigation," and the *Practical Homicide Investigation Checklist and Field Guide,* which is considered by professionals an essential prerequisite in conducting proficient death inquiries. Commander Geberth is also the author of *Sex-Related Homicide and Death Investigation: Practical and Clinical Perspectives,* Second Edition, which is considered the framework textbook on sex-related murder.

Commander Geberth is a nationally renowned lecturer, author, educator, consultant, and expert witness on the subject of death investigation. He has appeared on numerous local, national, and international television programs to answer questions on the subject of murder and provide insight, analysis, and commentary with respect to all aspects of homicide and death investigations. Geberth has been referenced as a media consultant on myriad national major cases across the United States and Canada. Over 65,000 members from over 8,000 law enforcement agencies have attended Geberth's Practical Homicide Investigation seminars.

In his seminars, Geberth focuses on advanced tactics, procedures, and forensic techniques and presents equivocal death, suicide, and missed investigations as well as serial murder investigation and the application of abnormal psychology to the investigative process.

Acknowledgments

First Name	Rank	Department/Agency
AAFS		American Academy of Forensic Science
Ronald Antonucci	Detective	Wayne Township, New Jersey, Police Department
Mark Benecke	Forensic scientist	International forensic research and consulting
Mark Burbridge	Detective	Spokane, Washington, Police Department
Terry Cousino	Detective	Toledo, Ohio, Police Department
Tom Cronin	Commander (ret.)	Chicago, Illinois, Police Department
Mark Czworniak	Detective	Chicago, Illinois, Police Department
Edward Dahlman	Detective	Columbus, Ohio Police Department
Edward Davies	Detective	Montgomery Township, Pennsylvania Police Department
Mark Fritts	Lieutenant (ret.)	New Mexico Police Department
Steve Gurka	Detective sergeant	Dearborn Heights, Michigan, Police Department
Krystal Gibson	Detective	Criminal Investigations Bureau, Knox County, Tennessee Sheriff's Office
Robert (Roy) Hazelwood	Supervisory special agent (ret.)	Federal Bureau of Investigation
Pete Farmer Hobbs	Sargeant (ret.)	New Mexico Police Department
Rich Kamholz	Detective	Rock County, Wisconsin, Sheriff's Department
Paul Koczwanski	Detective	Coventry, Rhode Island, Police Department
Raymond Krolak	Detective lieutenant (ret.)	Colonie, New York, Police Department
Steven Little	Detective	Columbus, Ohio, Police Department
Steve Mack	Detective (ret.)	Huntington Beach, California, Police Department
J. J. Mead	Detective, CSI	Columbus, Ohio, Police Department
Perry Meyers	Investigator	Lenexa, Kansas, Police Department
Scott Meyers	Detective	Coral Springs, Florida, Police Department
Mark Quagliarello	Detective	Raleigh, North Carolina, Police Department
Mark Reynolds	Detective sergeant	Harris County, Texas, Sheriff's Department
Robert Spoden	Sheriff	Rock County, Wisconsin, Sheriff's Department
David Vanderlpoeg	Sargeant	Village of Glenview, Illinois, Police Department
John J. Wiggins	Instructor–coordinator	North Carolina Criminal Justice Academy
Brian Wilson	Director of production	Medicolegal Art (MLA), Atlanta, Georgia

chapter one

Autoerotic death

Historical context

Sexual asphyxia in fiction

Long before becoming of forensic interest, erotic asphyxia had been described in fiction. The Marquis de Sade depicted erotic strangulation and hanging in his book *Justine*, published in 1791:

> He seizes my arms, binds them to my side, then he slips a black silken noose about my neck; he holds both ends of the cord and, by tightening, he can strangle and dispatch me to the other world either quickly or slowly, depending upon his pleasure. "This torture is sweeter than you may imagine, Therese," says Roland; "you will only approach death by way of unspeakably pleasurable sensations; the pressure this noose will bring to bear upon your nervous system will set fire to the organs of voluptuousness; the effect is certain. ... Therese, it's the rope that's waiting for me. ... I am as firmly persuaded as I can possibly be that this death is infinitely sweeter than cruel; but as the women upon whom I have tested its initial anguishes have never really wished to tell me the truth, it is in person I wish to be made acquainted with the sensation. By way of the experience itself I want to find out whether it is not very certain this asphyxiation impels, in the individual who undergoes it, the erectory nerve to produce an ejaculation; once convinced this death is but a game. ... You will do to me everything I did to you; I'll strip; I'll mount the stool, you'll adjust the rope, I'll excite myself for a moment, then, as soon as you see things assume a certain consistency, you'll jerk the stool free and I'll remain hanging; you'll leave me there until you either discern my semen's emission or symptoms of death's throes." ... We take our stations; Roland is stimulated by a few of his usual caresses; he climbs upon the stool, I put the halter round his neck. ... I do so; his dart soon rises to menace Heaven, he himself gives me the sign to remove the stool, I obey; would you believe it, Madame? nothing more true than what Roland had conjectured: nothing but symptoms of pleasure ornament his countenance and at practically the same instant rapid jets of semen spring nigh to the vault. When 'tis all shot out without any assistance whatsoever from me, I rush to cut him down, he falls, unconscious, but thanks to my ministrations he quickly recovers his senses. "Oh Therese!" he exclaims upon opening his eyes, "oh, those sensations are not to be described; they transcend all one can possibly say."

In 1833, in an anonymous book attributed to Alfred de Musset (*Gamiani ou Deux Nuits d'Excès*), a hanging is described that caused an erection in a previously sexually exhausted man. Jean Giono, another French author, portrayed the traditional autoerotic asphyxiation by a leather cowl among mountain people in the 19th century (*Faust au Village*).

Sexual hanging is also exposed in the German literature. At the beginning of the 20th century, Hanns Heinz Ewers wrote about sexual asphyxia in a book called *Alraune* and in a short story. In *Alraune*, a decadent law student blithely suggests that his wealthy scientist uncle artificially create a woman, as outlined in the legend of the fertility powers of the mandrake (or alraune) root. The uncle and the nephew collect the semen of a condemned murderer, ejaculated at the moment of hanging, and a prostitute is impregnated.

In the mid-20th century, there is an allusion to erection caused by hanging in the play *Waiting for Godot* by Samuel Beckett.

Vladimir: … What do we do?
Estragon: Wait.
Vladimir: Yes, but while waiting.
Estragon: What about hanging ourselves?
Vladimir: Hum. It'd give us an erection.
Estragon: (highly excited) An erection!
Vladimir: With all that follows. Where it falls mandrakes grow. That's why they shriek
  when you pull them up. Did you not know that?
Estragon: Let's hang ourselves immediately.

Anthropologists' accounts of autoerotic asphyxia

It is alleged that asphyxial games play a role in the sexuality of some other cultures. It seems that the Eskimos were known to choke each other as part of their sexual activity, and that it was common for their children to suspend themselves by the neck in playing games.[1] Similarly, it was alleged that the Yaghans of South America had asphyxial practices.[2] It has also been said that some Oriental lovers were grabbing each other's throat to enhance sexual pleasure.[3] However, it is rather difficult to distinguish myth from reality in these accounts.

The origin of autoerotic asphyxia in Western culture is not known. It is sometimes alleged that it might have come from the experiences of French Foreign Legionnaires who had been stationed in French Indochina (now Vietnam).

Sexual asphyxia: Early nonscientific reports in London

It is known that in the 17th century, prostitutes in London were using controlled strangulation as a cure for impotence and to enhance the pleasure of clients.[4,5]

Peter Anthony Motteux, a Huguenot refugee in London known for his completion of the translation of Rabelais's *Gargantua and Pantagruel* and his translation of Cervantes's *Don Quixote*, is probably the first recorded victim of autoerotic asphyxiation.[6] Though his death in 1718 was not considered sexually related at the time, a modern review of the case reveals that the man died in a London brothel of what seems to be assisted erotic asphyxia. Furthermore, an undated, unsigned marginal note in an old book on the lives of poets in the British library claimed, referring to Motteux, he "is suppos'd to have been strangled by Whores, who forgot to cut the cord They had ty'd abt his neck to provoke venery."[6]

Frantisek Kotzwara, a Czech composer known mainly for *The Battle of Prague*, is another early recorded victim of erotic asphyxiation.[5,7] On February 2, 1791, the same year as the publication of *Justine* by the Marquis de Sade, the musician visited a prostitute while in London. After dinner with her, it seems that Kotzwara paid her and requested that she cut off his testicles. The prostitute refused, and Kotzwara tied a ligature around the doorknob, fastened the other end around his neck, had sexual intercourse with the prostitute, and died. The prostitute, Susannah Hill, was subsequently tried for Kotzwara's murder, but the jury chose to believe her testimony, and she was acquitted. To avoid a public scandal, the court records of the case were ordered destroyed. It seems, however, that a copy was made and used to produce a pamphlet about the incident.

Historical context of autoerotic death in forensic literature

It is sometimes claimed that the earliest medical report of an autoerotic death is found in an old French monograph by de Boismont on suicide in 1856.[8] The sexual nature of the case, however, is not convincing: A 12-year-old boy was found hanging and, after being revived, stated that he had no desire to end his life but had a sudden urge to try to hang himself.

The early period (1947 to 1980)

In 1947, Simpson was the first to report a case in the United States*: "A naked youth was found in a lavatory hanging half off the edge of the seat, the penis turgid and dribbling semen, suspended from the neck by a rope to the inlet pipe of the cistern above. Several front page nudes from a picture newspaper were laid out in a half ring in front of him on the floor. Death was due to vagal inhibition and must have taken place suddenly, without warning. These cases must not be mistaken for suicides; they are accidental deaths."[9]

In 1953, Stearns brought to light a similar pattern in these bizarre deaths and suspected a syndrome related to masochism.[2] He described having observed one or two cases a year in Massachusetts between 1941 and 1950. From then, several cases started to be described. In 1957, Ford described six cases of autoerotic death,[10] followed in 1960 by four cases reported by Johnstone et al.,[11] and additional cases in 1963 by Usher.[12] In France, two cases were described by Van Hecke and Timperman.[13]

In 1960, Mant not only described three cases but also proposed criteria for the diagnosis[14]:

1. Evidence of asphyxia produced by strangulation, by either ligature or hanging, in which the position of the body, or the presence of protective measures such as padding about the neck, indicated that death was not obviously intended;
2. Evidence of sexual activity usually in the form of masturbation or perversion, especially Transvestism;
3. No well-defined evidence for suicide or minimal evidence of suicidal ideation or behavior;
4. Evidence of repetitive episodes.

---

* It seems that a sexual syndrome was described earlier in the German literature, starting in 1926, in a paper by Ziemke in *Archiv für Kriminologie* (78:262). The German literature was not accessible, however, to most forensic experts and remained unknown to them.

In 1967, Luke depicted his experience with hangings in New York City: Of 106 hanging deaths from 1964 to 1965, 2 were autoerotic hangings.[15] A series of seven more cases was published in 1970 by Gwozdz.[16]

In 1972, there were 25 cases reported in Los Angeles in the period 1958 to 1970.[17] The same year, Resnik proposed a new list of 10 criteria for the syndrome he called "erotized repetitive hanging(s)"[5]:

1. An adolescent or young adult male (it is in adolescence that the behavior begins; if the practitioner lives to adulthood, the syndrome can become less lethal as partners may become involved);
2. Ropes, belts or other binding material so arranged that compression of the neck may be produced and controlled voluntarily;
3. Evidence of masturbation (for example, semen);
4. Partial or complete nudity;
5. A solitary act;
6. Repetitive behavior that the deceased had tried to insure would leave no visible mark on his person;
7. No apparent wish to die;
8. The presence of erotic pictures or literature; and less frequently
9. Binding of the body and/or the extremities and/or genitals with ropes, chains or leather; and
10. Female attire may be present.

In 1971, the first female case was reported by Henry,[3] followed in 1975 and 1980 by two other female cases, described by Sass[18] and Danto.[19] Case reports of survivors also appeared in the 1970s.[17,20,21]

In 1977, the first study on the topic appeared[22]: A review of all deaths filed at the Armed Forces Institute of Pathology from 1958 to 1973 revealed 43 cases of autoerotic asphyxial deaths.

Despite these first attempts to define and understand autoerotic deaths, there was still no consensus or consistency on the label and definition of these deaths at the end of the 1970s.[23] Nevertheless, the syndrome was discussed in most forensic pathology textbooks by the end of that decade.[24–26]

The golden age (1981 to 1990)

In the 1980s, the number of reported cases exploded, and the syndrome became widely known. This golden age started with the publication in 1981 of the first study by Hazelwood et al.[23] Roy Hazelwood is one of the world's most famous profilers; he worked at the Behavioral Science Unit of the Federal Bureau of Investigation (FBI) Academy in Quantico, Virginia, for 16 years, until his retirement in 1994. He and Ann Wolbert Burgess, a nurse from the Boston University School of Nursing, collaborated on establishing the basis of the modern view of autoerotic deaths. Over a 1-year period, all trainees at the FBI Academy were briefed on autoerotic deaths and asked to send cases from their jurisdiction for the period 1970 to 1980. Seventy cases were collected. From the analyses of the data, five criteria were suggested:

1. Evidence of a physiological mechanism for obtaining or enhancing sexual arousal and dependent on either a self-rescue mechanism or the victim's judgment to discontinue its effect;
2. Evidence of solo sexual activity;

3. Evidence of sexual fantasy aids;
4. Evidence of prior dangerous autoerotic practice;
5. No apparent suicidal intent.

Hazelwood et al. in 1983 published the first book to present a comprehensive view of the topic.[27] It is in this book that they presented the incidence of 500 to 1,000 autoerotic deaths per year in the United States, a figure often cited currently. The same year, they published a study of 132 autoerotic asphyxial deaths notified by the Behavioral Science Unit of the FBI Academy.[28]

In the early period (1947 to 1980), autoerotic deaths were understood as hanging or ligature strangulation in a sexual context and less commonly as cases of asphyxia by plastic bags. In the golden age (1981 to 1990), other types of autoerotic asphyxia started to appear, such as autoerotic asphyxia by chemical substances.[29,30] The 1980s also witnessed the appearance of more bizarre autoerotic deaths, with case reports of electrocution,[31-33] body wrapping and overdressing,[34-36] drowning,[37] asphyxia by an abdominal ligature,[38] and death from foreign body insertion.[39,40] Unusual cases occurring outdoors also started to be described.[41,42]

Even though a few female cases were published in the early period, it was still thought that the usual criteria for the syndrome should be met. However, this conception changed after the publication of an important paper on female autoerotic death in 1988 by Byard and Bramwell.[43] The authors reported that the usual props present at the scene of male cases, such as pornographic material, female undergarments, and elaborate bizarre equipment, might not be as common in female cases. Based on this more subtle presentation, they suggested that female cases might be underdiagnosed. The comparative features of male and female autoerotic deaths were further explored in a later paper by Byard et al. in 1990.[44]

It was also during this period that awareness came about concerning the danger of exposing such phenomenon in the media. In 1988, O'Halloran and Lovell published a case of autoerotic death that happened shortly after the victim watched a television show discussing sexual asphyxia.[45] How individuals first learn of sexual asphyxia is still largely unknown. Although most people probably discover this sexual practice spontaneously, from word of mouth, or from pornography, the case of O'Halloran and Lovell made clear that media might play a role, and that forensic experts should be cautious in diffusing knowledge of this practice to the general population.

The turning point (1991)

In 1988, Imami and Kemal published a case of autoerotic death[46] that sparked a reaction from Byard and Bramwell.[47] The answer by Byard and Bramwell was a founding paper in the modern conception of autoerotic deaths and constituted a turning point in defining autoerotic deaths.

The case reported by Imami and Kemal was a 57-year-old white male discovered dead in his trailer home by a neighbor concerned by a continuously running vacuum cleaner.[46] The body was found naked, slumped over the vacuum cleaner on the dining room table. His testicles, thighs, and buttocks were bound with panty hose. A wooden table leg soiled with fecal material was also found at the scene, along with a bottle of wine, some food items, jars of lubricant, and a glass of urine. The wife stated that she once surprised the decedent masturbating with the vacuum cleaner. At autopsy, marked atherosclerotic coronary artery disease was documented. The cause of death was thought to be heart related, and the manner of death was ruled as natural, but in an autoerotic context. Byard and Bramwell answered in 1991 that the mere presence of unusual sexual props at a scene does not necessarily make a death autoerotic in nature.[47] They further stated that deaths from natural causes during unusual or bizarre autoerotic practice are not autoerotic deaths. The following definition, still in use, was proposed: Autoerotic deaths are accidental deaths that occur during individual, usually solitary, sexual activity in which a device, apparatus, or prop that was employed to enhance the sexual stimulation of the deceased in some way caused unintentional death. However, the term *sudden death during autoerotic practice* was proposed for natural deaths occurring during unusual or bizarre autoerotic practice.

Up to this turning point, the manner of death in autoerotic practice had been the subject of much discussion and controversy. Although over time more and more authors agreed that these deaths were accidental in nature, it was the paper of Byard and Bramwell that ended the debate.

The modern era

From 1991 to the present, multiple case reports have been published, mainly concerning unusual autoerotic methods or female cases. What is more characteristic of the modern era, however, is the emergence of systematic studies of autoerotic deaths. Before 1991, apart from the studies by Hazelwood et al., studies were virtually nonexistent. In the modern era, several studies were published: a study of 117 cases by Blanchard and Hucher,[48] a 57-year study by Behrendt and Modvig,[49] a 20-year study by Breitmeier et al.,[50] another 20-year study by Janssen et al.,[51] and a 9-year study by Shields et al.[52]

Another important landmark in the history of forensic literature on autoerotic deaths was an article in 2006 reviewing all published cases from 1954 to 2004.[53] Based on this review, the methods of autoerotic deaths were classified as typical or atypical. Typical methods include hangings, ligatures, plastic bags, chemical substances, and mixtures of these. Atypical methods leading to death are electrocution, overdressing/body wrapping, foreign body insertion, atypical asphyxia method, and miscellaneous. The typical and atypical methods are discussed further in Chapters 4 through 6.

The need for a modern book covering the advances on autoerotic death

Despite the advances in the knowledge of autoerotic death since the golden age, the most comprehensive book on autoerotic death remained *Autoerotic Fatalities*, published in 1983 by Hazelwood et al.[27] The present book aims at filling this gap by providing a comprehensive modern view of autoerotic deaths.

References

1. Freuchen P. *Book of the Eskimos*. Cleveland, OH: World, 1961.
2. Stearns AW. Cases of probable suicide in young persons without obvious motivation. *J Maine Med Assoc* 1953;44(1):16–23.
3. Henry RD. *Medico-Legal Bulletin*. Office of the Chief Medical Examiner, Department of Health, State of Virginia, 1971;20(2):Bulletin 214.
4. Rosenblum S, Faber MM. The adolescent sexual asphyxia syndrome. *J Am Acad Child Psychiatry* 1979;18(3):546–558.

5. Resnik HL. Erotized repetitive hangings: a form of self-destructive behaviour. *Am J Psychother* 1972;26(1):4–21.

6. Ober WB. The man in the scarlet cloak. The mysterious death of Peter Anthony Motteux. *Am J Forensic Med Pathol* 1991;12(3):255–261.

7. Ober WB. The sticky end of Frantisek Koczwara, composer of "The Battle of Prague." *Am J Forensic Med Pathol* 1984;5(2):145–149.

8. de Boismont AB. *Du Suicide et de la Folie Suicide*. Paris: Germer Bailliere, 1856.

9. Simpson K. *Forensic Medicine*. Baltimore: Williams and Wilkins, 1947.

10. Ford R. Death by hanging of adolescent and young adult males. *Forensic Sci* 1957;2:171.

11. Johnstone JM, Hunt AC, Ward EM. Plastic-bag asphyxia in adults. *Br Med J* 1960;2(5214):1714–1715.

12. Usher A. Accidental hanging in relation to abnormal sexual practices. *Newcastle Med J* 1963;27:234–237.

13. Van Hecke W, Timperman J. [Hanging as the cause of accidental death in an unusual form of sex perversion. Report of two cases] [In French]. *Ann Med Leg Criminol Police Sci Toxicol* 1963;43:218–222.

14. Mant AK. *Forensic Medicine*. Chicago: Year Book, 1960:113–127.

15. Luke JL. Asphyxial deaths by hanging in New York City, 1964–1965. *J Forensic Sci* 1967;12(3):359–369.

16. Gwozdz F. The sexual asphyxia: review of current concepts and presentation of seven cases. *Forensic Sci Gazette* 1970:1(1):24.

17. Litman RE, Swearingen C. Bondage and suicide. *Arch Gen Psychiatry* 1972;27(1):81–85.

18. Sass FA. Sexual asphyxia in the female. *Forensic Sci* 1975;20(1):181–185.

19. Danto BL. A case of female autoerotic death. *Am J Forensic Med Pathol* 1980;1(2):117–121.

20. Edmondson JS. A case of sexual asphyxia without fatal termination. *Br J Psychiatry* 1972;121:437–438.

21. Herman SP. Recovery from hanging in an adolescent male. *Clin Pediatr* 1974;13:854–856.

22. Walsh FM, Stahl CJ, 3rd, Unger HT, Lilienstern OC, Stephens RG, 3rd. Autoerotic asphyxial deaths: a medicolegal analysis of forty-three cases. *Leg Med Ann* 1977;155–182.

23. Hazelwood RR, Burgess AW, Groth N. Death during dangerous autoerotic practice. *Soc Sci Med* 1981;15:129–133.

24. Polson CJ, Gee DJ. *The Essentials of Forensic Medicine*. Oxford, UK: Pergamon Press, 1973.

25. Camps FE, ed. *Gradwohl's Legal Medicine*, 3rd edition. Bristol, UK: Wright, 1976.

26. Simpson K. *Forensic Medicine*, 8th edition. London: Arnold, 1979.

27. Hazelwood RR, Dietz PE, Burgess AW, eds. *Autoerotic Fatalities*. Lexington, MA: Lexington Books, Heath, 1983.

28. Burgess AW, Hazelwood RR. Autoerotic asphyxial deaths and social network response. *Am J Orthopsychiatry* 1983;53(1):166–170.

29. Cordner SM. An unusual case of sudden death associated with masturbation. *Med Sci Law* 1983;23(1):54–56.

30. Leadbeatter S. Dental anesthetic death. An unusual autoerotic episode. *Am J Forensic Med Pathol* 1988;9(1):60–63.

31. Cairns FJ. Death from electrocution during auto-erotic procedures. *N Z Med J* 1981;94(693):259–260.

32. Sivaloganathan S. Curiosum eroticum—a case of fatal electrocution during auto-erotic practice. *Med Sci Law* 1981;21(1):47–50.

33. Tan CTT, Chao TC. A case of fatal electrocution during an unusual auto-erotic practice. *Med Sci Law* 1983;23(2):92–95.

34. Eriksson A, Gezelius C, Bring G. Rolled up to death. *Am J Forensic Med Pathol* 1987;8(3):263–265.

35. Minyard F. Wrapped to death. Unusual autoerotic death. *Am J Forensic Med Pathol* 1985;6(2):151–152.

36. Ikeda N, Harada A, Umetsu K, Suzuki T. A case of fatal suffocation during an unusual auto-erotic practice. *Med Sci Law* 1988;28(2):131–134.

37. Sivaloganathan S. Aqua-eroticum—a case of auto-erotic drowning. *Med Sci Law* 1984;24(4):300–302.

38. Thibault R, Spencer JD, Bishop JW, Hibler NS. An unusual autoerotic death: asphyxia with an abdominal ligature. *J Forensic Sci* 1984;29(2):679–684.

39. Sivaloganathan S. Catheteroticum. Fatal late complication following autoerotic practice. *Am J Forensic Med Pathol* 1985;6(4):340–342.

40. Marc B, Chadly A, Durigon M. Fatal air embolism during female autoerotic practice. *Int J Leg Med* 1990;104:59–61.

41. Emson HE. Accidental hanging in autoeroticism. An unusual case occurring outdoors. *Am J Forensic Med Pathol* 1983;4(4):337–340.

42. Hiss J, Rosenberg SB, Adelson L. "Swinging in the park." An investigation of an autoerotic death. *Am J Forensic Med Pathol* 1985;6(3):250–255.

43. Byard RW, Bramwell NH. Autoerotic death in females. An underdiagnosed syndrome? *Am J Forensic Med Pathol* 1988;9(2):252–254.

44. Byard RW, Hucker SJ, Hazelwood RR. A comparison of typical death scene features in cases of fatal male and female autoerotic asphyxia with a review of the literature. *Forensic Sci Int* 1990;48(2):113–121.

45. O'Halloran RL, Lovell FW. Autoerotic asphyxial death following television broadcast. *J Forensic Sci* 1988;33(6):1491–1492.

46. Imami RH, Kemal M. Vacuum cleaner use in autoerotic death. *Am J Forensic Med Pathol* 1988;9:246–248.

47. Byard RW, Bramwell NH. Autoerotic death—a definition. *Am J Forensic Med Pathol* 1991;12(1):74–76.

48. Blanchard R, Hucker SJ. Age, transvestism, bondage, and concurrent paraphilic activities in 117 fatal cases of autoerotic asphyxia. *Br J Psychiatry* 1991;159:371–377.

49. Behrendt N, Modvig J. The lethal paraphilic syndrome. Accidental autoerotic deaths in Denmark 1933–1990. *Am J Forensic Med Pathol* 1995;16(3):232–237.

50. Breitmeier D, Mansorui F, Albrecht K, et al. Accidental autoerotic deaths between 1978 and 1997. Institute of Legal Medicine, Medical School Hannover. *Forensic Sci Int* 2003;137(1):41–44.

51. Janssen W, Koops E, Anders S, et al. Forensic aspects of 40 accidental autoerotic deaths in northern Germany. *Forensic Sci Int* 2005;147:Suppl S61–S64.

52. Shields LB, Hunsaker DM, Hunsaker JC, 3rd. Autoerotic asphyxia: part I. *Am J Forensic Med Pathol* 2005;26(1):45–52.

53. Sauvageau A, Racette S. Autoerotic death in the literature from 1954 to 2004: A review. *J Forensic Sci* 2006;51(1):140–146.

chapter two

Definition, incidence, and best practices in approaching these deaths

Definition

The most widely used definition of *autoerotic death* is the one by Byard and Bramwell, formulated in 1991: Autoerotic deaths are accidental deaths that occur during individual, usually solitary, sexual activity in which some type of apparatus that was used to enhance the sexual stimulation of the deceased caused unintentional death.[1]

This definition was put forward in response to a case that was published by Imami and Kemal in 1988.[2] A 57-year-old man was found dead, naked, slumped over a vacuum cleaner on a dining room table. His testicles, thighs, and buttocks were bound with panty hose. The man was masturbating with the vacuum cleaner when he suffered a heart attack and died. That case was reported as an autoerotic death based on the unusual associated props at the scene (vacuum cleaner, panty hose, jar of lubricant, glass of urine, wooden table leg with fecal material). As pointed out by Byard and Bramwell in their answer of 1991, this case of Imami and Kemal was a natural death occurring during masturbation, and that such cases should not be called autoerotic deaths.[2] Their definition, in reaction to this case, contains two important elements that are still of great importance: The manner of death in autoerotic death should always be accidental, and death should be directly linked to the use of an apparatus for sexual stimulation.

From a modern perspective, the definition of Byard and Bramwell is still accurate overall but needs to be modified on one important aspect: Autoerotic deaths are not *usually* solitary but *always* solitary. The term *autoerotic* comes from the Greek root *auto*, which means self or by itself. Therefore, an autoerotic death that is not solitary is a contradiction of terms. Cases in which asphyxial games or other sexual games with a partner in some way caused death of one of the protagonists are not autoerotic deaths. They are accidental deaths in a sexual context, but not autoerotic.

The best definition for autoerotic deaths is the following: Autoerotic deaths are accidental deaths that occur during solitary sexual activity in which some type of apparatus that was used to enhance the sexual stimulation of the deceased caused unintentional death.

Pitfalls in the application of the term autoerotic death

In our experience, there are three pitfalls commonly encountered in the application of the term *autoerotic death*. These errors are surprisingly widespread, even among the forensic community. We have encountered cases of these errors committed by otherwise highly competent forensic pathologists. One of us has sadly had to reject papers during the peer review process for forensic journals because of accumulation of these basic mistakes in a single paper. These widespread pitfalls are as follows:

1. To label a death autoerotic even though the manner of death was not accidental
2. To label a death autoerotic even though the sexual activity was not solitary
3. To become confused concerning the concept of an escape mechanism

Pitfall 1: To label a death autoerotic even though the manner of death was not accidental

By definition, autoerotic deaths are always accidental deaths. If the manner of death is ruled as natural, suicide, homicide, or undetermined, then the case cannot be labeled an autoerotic death.

A man suffering a heart attack (myocardial infarction) during masturbation did not have an autoerotic death. Other types of natural deaths, such as by a rupture of a cerebral aneurysm or a dissection of the aorta, are not autoerotic deaths, even if the scene is rich in sexual elements. Sexual activity, as exercising, has important cardiovascular effects that can increase the risk of certain types of sudden death. For example, the risk of cardiac death and death by rupture of a cerebral aneurysm are known to be increased by sexual activity. Despite a possible link in the cause of death and the sexual activity, such cases cannot be ruled as autoerotic deaths since the manner of death was natural. There is no exception to this rule. Even a death in an elaborate scene of autoerotic activity, with bondage, various masochistic features, cross-dressing, and a mirror cannot be called an autoerotic death if the final cause of death is found at autopsy to be a myocardial infarction or another type of natural death. The manner of death in autoerotic death cannot be natural, without exception.

Suicide cases also cannot be labeled autoerotic deaths. The absence of evidence of suicidal intent constitutes one of the mandatory criteria for ruling a death as autoerotic. For example, if a naked man with bondage of the genitals was found dead hanging, the presence of a suicidal letter at the scene would avert the case from being called autoerotic unless there is evidence that the letter was left at the scene by a third party in an attempt to conceal the true nature of the death.

Pitfall 2: To label a death autoerotic even though the sexual activity was not solitary

By definition, autoerotic deaths have to be secondary to a solitary sexual activity. To call *auto* a death that occurs during an activity with a partner is an oxymoron. The deaths of victims killed inadvertently during consensual sexual games cannot be called autoerotic deaths. The same is true of unwilling victims killed in the context of the sexual fantasy of their aggressor.

Pitfall 3: To become confused concerning the concept of an escape mechanism

In the historical development of the concept of autoerotic death, one of the key events was the publication in 1981 of a study by Hazelwood et al.[3] This publication marked the beginning of the golden age (1981–1990) of autoerotic deaths in the forensic literature (see Chapter 1). Roy Hazelwood was a profiler at the Behavioral Science Unit of the Federal Bureau of Investigation (FBI) Academy in Quantico, Virginia, and he worked closely with Ann Wolbert Burgess, a nurse from the Boston University School of Nursing. Their 1981 study was based on a 1-year survey of all trainees at the FBI Academy. After being briefed on autoerotic deaths, trainees were asked to send cases from their jurisdiction for the period 1970 to 1980. Seventy cases were collected, and from the analyses of the data, criteria for determining death as autoerotic were suggested. Among these criteria was the following: evidence of a physiological mechanism for obtaining or enhancing sexual arousal and dependent on either a self-rescue mechanism or the victim's judgment to discontinue its effect.

The intent of the autoerotic practitioner is not to die. The practitioner has an idea of how to get out of the dangerous situation to ensure survival. To do so, the practitioner sometimes uses a rescue mechanism. For example, a chair positioned near a hanging point can allow the practitioner to release the tension on the neck by simply standing on the chair. For example, in a case of autoerotic asphyxia by drowning published by Sivaloganathan, a man was using water submersion as a sexual enhancer, plunging in the water with a large stone tied to his ankles by a clothesline.[4] When he had reached a level of asphyxia that he considered enough, he would cut the clothesline with a pair of scissors. Rescue mechanisms can be as simple as these examples of the chair and scissors or can be quite elaborate.

In the vast majority of cases, however, there is no self-rescue mechanism. Some then make the mistake of assuming that in the absence of a distinct self-rescue mechanism at the scene, the death cannot be called autoerotic. They are forgetting that, as correctly pointed out by Hazelwood et al.,[3] the practitioner can also rely on personal judgment to discontinue the dangerous activity instead of using a tangible self-rescue. In fact, in our experience, there is no concrete self-rescue mechanism found in the majority of autoerotic death scenes. The practitioner will hang himself, for example, from a kneeling position and will control the pressure on his neck by leaning forward to increase the asphyxia or backward to release it. Or, he will hang himself from a standing position, feet on the ground, and will control the pressure on the neck by flexing or extending his legs. In asphyxia by plastic bag or chemical substances, the practitioner will remove the bag or discontinue the gas exposure.

Case history: Typical autoerotic death—outdoor secluded location

One of us had the occasion to review an autoerotic case for which at first the medical examiner did not want to rule the case accidental–autoerotic because there was no escape mechanism to the noose. The medical examiner was under the impression that there had to be an escape mechanism to have an autoerotic death classification. The investigator showed the medical examiner a copy the textbook *Practical Homicide Investigation,* which illustrated that often there is not an escape mechanism, just bad judgment.

The victim, a male, white, 53 years of age, was reported missing by his wife when he failed to come home from work at a nursery. Uniform officers located the victim's car at his place of work and conducted a ground and aerial search of the large 1-square-mile nursery grounds.

A triangulation by the cell phone provider indicated that his phone was within 150 meters of the search area. The victim's body was found hanging in a secret room behind his workstation at the nursery (Figures 2.1 and 2.2). The victim had constructed a private place that even his coworkers were not aware of until his body was found. He was on his knees hanging from a noose that was attached to some piping, which ran across the ceiling. There was also another, older noose hanging from the same pipe. The victim was nude, his armpits were shaved, and he had nail polish on his toes (Figures 2.3 and 2.4). Investigators recovered numerous items of female lingerie (panties, stockings, and a slip), a woman's wig, makeup, and a whip and ball gag (Figure 2.5). Interviews of the man's wife indicated that he had become involved in kinky masturbation practices with pornography and had even hooked his penis to a car battery while engaging in solo sexual activities.

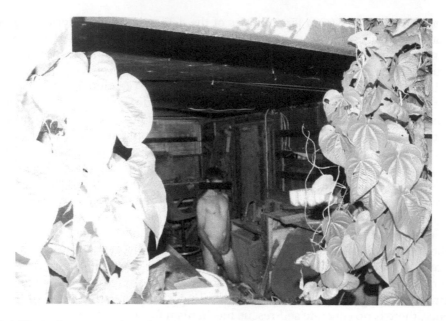

Figure 2.1 Victim hanging in kneeling position. (Courtesy of Detective Scott Myers, Coral Springs, Florida, Police Department; submitted from author Geberth's files.)

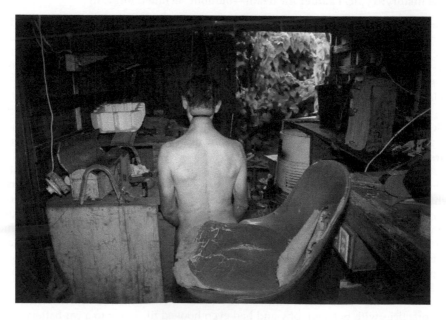

Figure 2.2 Rear view of victim. (Courtesy of Detective Scott Myers, Coral Springs, Florida, Police Department; submitted from author Geberth's files.)

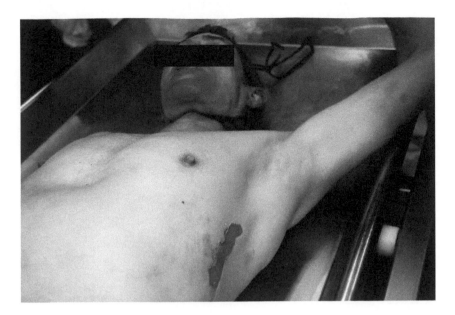

Figure 2.3 Shaved armpits. (Courtesy of Detective Scott Myers, Coral Springs, Florida, Police Department; submitted from author Geberth's files.)

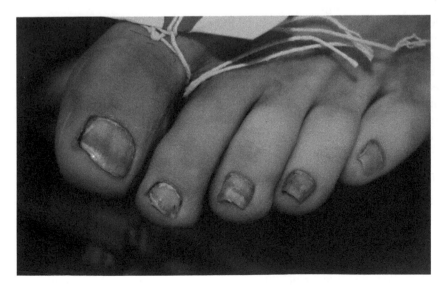

Figure 2.4 Nail polish on toes. (Courtesy of Detective Scott Myers, Coral Springs, Florida, Police Department; submitted from author Geberth's files.)

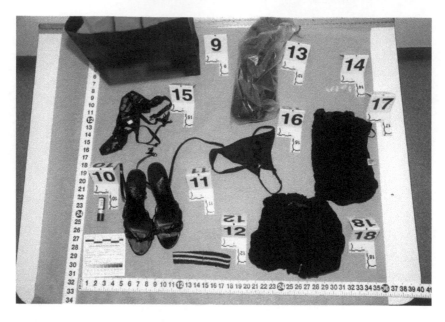

Figure 2.5 Women's lingerie recovered from scene. (Courtesy of Detective Scott Myers, Coral Springs, Florida, Police Department; submitted from author Geberth's files.)

Terminology and death certification

Over time, different terms have been used to refer to autoerotic deaths: sex hanging, masochistic hanging, masturbatory fatalities, hypoxyphilia, hypoxyphilic behavior, asphyxiophilia, autoerotic asphyxial death, autoerotic asphyxia, sexual asphyxia, autoerotic suicide, sexual bondage suicide, terminal sex, suicide without motivation, Kotzwarraism. Several of these terms are inappropriate and misleading. Some are too restrictive, and some are not precise enough.

To designate these deaths as a whole, the best term is autoerotic death. It is strongly recommended to avoid the term *autoerotic asphyxia* when referring to all types of autoerotic fatalities since some autoerotic deaths are not related to asphyxia (e.g., autoerotic electrocution). The term *autoerotic death* is more accurate.

In certifying death, it is recommended to use the term *autoerotic* in association with the method of autoeroticism that accidently caused death. For example, the cause of death can be autoerotic hanging or autoerotic electrocution. The manner of death should always be ruled accidental.

Incidence of autoerotic deaths

The incidence of autoerotic deaths is widely cited in the literature as around 500 to 1,000 deaths per year in the United States. This incidence originated from a book by Hazelwood et al. in 1983,[5] later cited in an article by Burgess and Hazelwood.[6] Until recently, this incidence of 500 to 1,000 cases per year in the United States was of general acceptance. A recent article, however, pointed out two important problems with this incidence.[7]

First, this alleged incidence of 500 to 1,000 deaths per year in the United States is based on data from 1983. Since that time, the population in the United States has increased significantly. Considering that the population of the United States in 1983 was 226.5 million[8] and reached 309 million in 2010,[9] the estimate of Hazelwood et al. should now be 700 to 1,400 deaths per year.

There is also a more serious problem with continuing to cite these data as fact: Contrary to the general assumption, Hazelwood and his team never conducted a study. Most forensic experts who cite the incidence of 500 to 1,000 cases per year never read the original source in the 1983 book and simply assumed that a study had been conducted. Here is the extract concerning the origin of the alleged incidence of 500 to 1,000 autoerotic deaths per year in the United States:

> Sir David Paul, coroner for the City of London, estimated that there were 4 deaths per year in a population at risk of over 2 million. Unpublished data from Ontario, Canada, suggest an incidence of approximately 1 death per million population per year (courtesy of Dr. S. Hucker, Clarke Institute, University of Toronto). If the incidence of detected and reported cases is, in fact, 1 to 2 deaths per million population per year, and if we assume that approximately half of cases are detected and reported, the actual number of cases occurring in the United-States could be estimated at 500 to 1,000 per year. Such estimates, however, are highly speculative because both the reported incidence and the percentage of cases are unknown.[5]

Hazelwood et al. never conducted an epidemiological study. They only guesstimated an incidence based on unpublished estimates from other countries. Since this estimation of the number of autoerotic deaths per year in the United States by comparison with Canada and United Kingdom was made, no epidemiological studies have been conducted in the United States.

In 2008, a Canadian study directly challenged this estimate.[10] The comments on the article were virulent: How could someone dare to challenge the great study of Hazelwood et al.? It was alleged by the detractors of the article that the observed difference was not a proof of the invalidity of the incidence found by Hazelwood et al. but instead could be easily explained by a Canadian–United States divergence in incidence.

The criticisms expressed in this chapter are not criticism of the book of Hazelwood et al., who did the best they could with the available material at the time. The criticism is toward us as a forensic community: We should be careful when attributing a gold value to a source, either an article or a book, and should have taken the basic precaution to have read the source and evaluated the true value of this alleged unchallengeable piece of knowledge. No book or article should ever become a forever bible as science is not a religion and should never stop evolving.

Having established that the incidence of 500 to 1,000 autoerotic deaths per year in United States is of limited current value, we can now look at the available epidemiological studies worldwide.

Incidence in Canada

In the province of Quebec (Canada), a 7-year study from 2000 to 2006 found only 9 cases in a population of 7.5 million, corresponding to an incidence of 0.2 cases per million inhabitants per year.[10] In comparison, 500 to 1,000 deaths per year in the United States in 1983 (population of 226.5 million) was reckoned with an incidence of 2.2 to 4.4 cases per million inhabitants per year. In other words, if the estimate of Hazelwood et al.[5] was valid, 115 to

231 cases should have been found in the 7-year study in the province of Quebec, whereas only 9 cases were actually found.

Blanchard and Hucker reviewed all death certificates for autoerotic deaths from 1974 to 1987 in the provinces of Ontario and Alberta.[11] A total of 117 cases was found, corresponding to approximately 0.75 cases per million inhabitants per year.

Another Canadian study conducted in the province of Alberta found 38 autoerotic deaths in a 25-year period (1985 to 2009), for an incidence of 0.56 cases per million inhabitants per year.[7]

Incidence in Europe

The incidence of 0.2 to 0.5 autoerotic deaths per million inhabitants per year in Canada is in keeping with several European studies. In Germany, 11 cases were found in the Hannover region from 1978 to 1997, representing an incidence of 0.49 cases per million inhabitants per year,[12] whereas 40 cases were found in Hamburg from 1983 to 2003, representing an incidence of 0.5 cases per million inhabitants per year.[13] In other studies, the incidence was 0.1 cases per million inhabitants per year in Sweden,[14] 0.5 in Denmark,[15] and 0.5 to 1 in Scandinavia.[16]

Incidence of autoerotic deaths in Western Countries

It seems that the incidence of autoerotic deaths in Western countries varies from 0.2 to 1 per million inhabitants per year, with an average of approximately 0.5. In the United States, this incidence corresponds to about 155 cases per year.

Although no American study is available, an incidence can be grossly calculated from two previous studies in Kentucky.[17,18] It seems that in this state, there were 20 cases of autoerotic deaths from 1993 to 2001 (16 autoerotic asphyxia and 4 atypical cases). Considering the population of Kentucky to be about 4 million during this period,[19] the incidence was of 0.55 cases per million inhabitants per year. This is in keeping with the estimated 0.5 cases per million per year.

Variables influencing the incidence of autoerotic deaths

Even though the incidence of autoerotic deaths seems rather similar throughout Western countries, it is probable cultural and socioeconomic factors play a role. In a recent Canadian study, it was demonstrated that Calgary had a higher incidence (0.76) compared to Edmonton (0.57) and to the rest of Alberta (0.44).[7] According to this study, urban areas might have a higher incidence than rural areas, and bigger cities with white-collar lifestyle might have a higher incidence than smaller, blue-collar cities. Further research is needed to better define cultural and socioeconomic factors contributing to the incidence of these deaths.

Best practices in approaching these deaths

In the investigation of these deaths (as well as in the investigation of almost all other types of deaths), the forensic expert must consider all aspects of the golden triangle of forensic investigation: a complete analysis of the scene, the examination of the body, and the history (past medical history, psychiatric history, sexual history, etc.) (Figure 2.6). There is an interdependence of all the evidence, and none of these elements can be interpreted

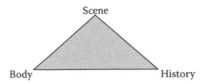

Figure 2.6 The golden triangle of forensic investigation.

separately. Each of these elements is equally important. Without this integrated approach, homicides could be missed, or suicides and natural deaths could be misinterpreted as autoerotic accidents.

Investigation of the scene

The typical autoerotic death scene usually presents a rich mixture of the following characteristics: nudity or exposed genitals, cross-dressing, pornography, mirror or video recording, bondage, and other masochistic elements. The scene characteristics are discussed further in Chapter 3. It is important that no suicide letter is found at the scene.

In female cases, there are usually few scene elements to be found. This paucity of scenic elements and the most useful clues to avoid missing the female cases are addressed in Chapter 7.

Examination of the body

A proper examination of the body should be conducted in every case. The following basic characteristics should be documented: height and weight, hair length and color, color of the eyes, natural teeth or not, tattoos, scars, any other distinctive signs. Clothing should be documented. Livor mortis and rigor mortis should be commented on, along with a comment if there are signs of decomposition present. All injuries should be properly documented.

The other elements that are of importance during the examination of the body (either external examination or autopsy) will vary depending on the type of autoerotic death. The external examination and autopsy findings are further discussed in Chapter 4 (hanging), Chapter 5 (suffocation by plastic bags and chemical substances), and Chapter 6 (atypical autoerotic methods).

History

The investigator needs to perform a complete history investigation, including a medical history, a psychiatric history, and a sexual history. One point is of tremendous importance in the history investigation: There should be no evidence of suicidal ideation. If there are some concerns that suicide is a probable manner of death, it would be better to avoid labeling the death as autoerotic accidental death. In such instances, it is better to rule the manner as either suicide or undetermined, depending on the degree of probability that death is indeed a suicide, and not to use the term *autoerotic* in certifying death.

Often in autoerotic death, close friends or family members will report a past sexual history of interest to interpret the death as autoerotic. For example, it is common to have a history that the decedent was surprised during solitary sexual activity of a similar nature. A father would have gone to the basement and found his son playing with hanging himself. Or, a mother will say that she noticed a broken shower rod a few weeks before the decedent was found hanged from a shower rod in the same bathroom.

Sexual partners, present and past, are of high interest for the investigation of the sexual history. Often, the decedent will have asked his partner to participate in sexual activities with some similarities with the fatal event. A sexual partner could mention that the decedent used to ask to be partially strangulated during sexual intercourse (these individuals would usually say "choked" even though it is a misnomer) or that the decedent liked to use bondage, and the bondage described could be highly similar to that observed at the fatal event.

An investigation of the content of the decedent's personal computer is also often informative. The decedent will often have consulted websites of similar sexual practices, will be found to have been a member of associations or groups of people sharing similar sexual interest or practices, or will be found to have written concerning his own sexual fantasies or experiences on social media networks, message boards, or chat rooms.

Understanding these deaths: There are different types of sexuality

One of the most difficult parts of the investigation is often to understand how some of these deaths are sexual in nature. To do so, the forensic expert has to remember that there are three general sources of sexual pleasure: stimulation of the genital organs, lack of oxygen in the central nervous system, and the creation of an atmosphere of fear and anguish in the context of masochism.

For the vast majority of people, their sexual pleasure is mainly related to the direct stimulation of the genital organs. For other people, the lack of oxygen to the brain is a sexual activity in itself. It is well known that a lack of oxygen to the brain can create intense sexual pleasure. At first, the asphyxia will often be combined with masturbation or sexual intercourse, but over time, the need to masturbate at the same time will decrease, and the asphyxia itself becomes the sexual activity. Similarly, the creation of a context of fear and anguish is a source of intense sexual pleasure for some individuals. These masochistic behaviors can be combined with direct genital stimulation or asphyxia or can become the sexual activity itself.

It is important to understand that evidence of masturbation during the autoerotic fatal event is not mandatory. On the contrary, it is rare that such evidence will be found. The presence of semen does not necessarily indicate prior masturbation since it is well known that postmortem ejaculation can occur.

Definition of autoerotic deaths: Checklist for the forensic expert

- Define autoerotic deaths as accidental deaths that occur during solitary sexual activity in which some type of apparatus that was used to enhance the sexual stimulation of the deceased caused unintentional death.
- Be aware of the three pitfalls in the application of the term autoerotic:
  1. Never label a death autoerotic if the manner is not accidental.
  2. Never label a death autoerotic if the sexual activity is not solitary.
  3. Know that an escape mechanism is not mandatory for labeling a death autoerotic.
- Do not use the terms *autoerotic death* and *autoerotic asphyxia* as synonyms.
- In certifying death, use the term *autoerotic* in association with the method of autoeroticism (e.g., autoerotic hanging).
- In certifying death, always rule the manner as accidental in autoerotic deaths.

Incidence of autoerotic deaths: Checklist for the forensic expert

- Do not cite an incidence of 500 to 1,000 autoerotic deaths per year in the United States.
- Cite an incidence of approximately 0.5 autoerotic deaths per million inhabitants per year.
- Be aware that cities seem to have a higher incidence than rural areas.
- Be aware that cultural and socioeconomic factors might play a role in the incidence.

Best approaches of autoerotic deaths: Checklist for the forensic expert

- Be aware that all elements of the golden triangle of investigation are equally important: scene, body, and history.
- Always conduct a complete scene investigation, proper examination of the body, and complete history investigation before ruling death as an autoerotic accidental death.

Understanding these deaths: There are different types of sexuality

- Understand that direct stimulation of the genital organs is not the only possible source of pleasure for certain individuals.
- Know that masturbation is not a mandatory element of autoerotic death.

References

1. Byard RW, Bramwell NH. Autoerotic death—a definition. *Am J Forensic Med Pathol* 1991;12(1):74–76.
2. Imami RH, Kemal M. Vacuum cleaner use in autoerotic death. *Am J Forensic Med Pathol* 1988;9:246–248.
3. Hazelwood RR, Burgess AW, Groth N. Death during dangerous autoerotic practice. *Soc Sci Med* 1981;15:129–133.
4. Sivaloganathan S. Aqua-eroticum—a case of auto-erotic drowning. *Med Sci Law* 1984;24(4):300–302.
5. Hazelwood RR, Dietz PE, Burgess AW. Asphyxial autoerotic fatalities. In: Hazelwood RR, Dietz PE, Burgess AW (eds.), *Autoerotic Fatalities*. Lexington, MA: Books, Heath, 1983:55–76.
6. Burgess AW, Hazelwood RR. Autoerotic asphyxial deaths and social network response. *Am J Orthopsychiatry* 1983;53(1):166–170.
7. Sauvageau A. Autoerotic deaths: a 25-year retrospective epidemiological study. *Am J Forensic Med Pathol* 2012;33(2):143–146.
8. Hobbs F, Stoops N. *U.S. Census Bureau. Demographic Trends in the 20th Century*. Census 2000 Special Reports, Series CENSR-4. Washington, DC: U.S. Government Printing Office, 2002.
9. U.S. Census Bureau. U.S. and world population clocks. http://www.census.gov/main/www/popclock.html (accessed April 12, 2010).
10. Sauvageau A. Autoerotic deaths: a retrospective epidemiological study. *Open Forensic Sci J* 2008;1:1–3.
11. Blanchard R, Hucker SJ. Age, transvestism, bondage, and concurrent paraphilic activities in 117 fatal cases of autoerotic asphyxia. *Br J Psychiatry* 1991;159:371–377.
12. Breitmeier D, Mansorui F, Albrecht K, et al. Accidental autoerotic deaths between 1978 and 1997. Institute of Legal Medicine, Medical School Hannover. *Forensic Sci Int* 2003;137(1):41–44.
13. Janssen W, Koops E, Anders S, et al. Forensic aspects of 40 accidental autoerotic deaths in northern Germany. *Forensic Sci Int* 2005;147:Suppl S61–S64.

14. Flobecker P, Ottoson J, Johansson L, Hietala M-A, Gezelius C, Eriksson A. Accidental deaths from asphyxia, a 10-year retrospective study from Sweden. *Am J Forensic Med Pathol* 1993;14(1):74–80.
15. Behrendt N, Modvig J. The lethal paraphilic syndrome. Accidental autoerotic deaths in Denmark 1933–1990. *Am J Forensic Med Pathol* 1995;16(3):232-37.
16. Innala SM, Ernulf KE. Asphyxiophilia in Scandinavia. *Arch Sex Behav* 1989;18(3):181–189.
17. Shields LB, Hunsaker DM, Hunsaker JC, 3rd. Autoerotic asphyxia: part I. *Am J Forensic Med Pathol* 2005;26(1):45–52.
18. Shields LB, Hunsaker DM, Hunsaker JC, 3rd, Wetli CV, Hutchins KD, Holmes RM. Atypical autoerotic death: part II. *Am J Forensic Med Pathol* 2005;26(1):53–62.
19. U.S. Census Bureau, Population Division. Population. http://www.google.com/publicdata?ds=uspopulation&met=population&idim=state:21000&dl=en&hl=en&q=kentucky+population (accessed April 12, 2010).

chapter three

Death scene characteristics

Death scene characteristics as main clues to the sexual autoerotic nature

The autoerotic nature of a death is mainly established by the death scene. Several features are commonly observed at the scene of autoerotic deaths: nudity or exposed genitals, cross-dressing, pornography, mirror or video recording, bondage, evidence of masochistic behavior, protective padding in hanging cases, evidence of masturbatory activity, and evidence of repetitive behavior. These various scene characteristics constitute clues to the accidental nature of the sexually related death. Regardless of the autoerotic method used (e.g., hanging, chemical gases, electrocution), the investigation team is led in the direction of an accidental autoerotic death by the presence of these characteristics at the scene.

In fact, the crime scene characteristics are more useful to establish the autoerotic nature of a death than the autoerotic method. Not only are the autoerotic methods encountered diverse, but also none of these methods is specific for autoerotic deaths. For example, the most common method of autoerotic death is hanging. However, most hangings are not autoerotic accidents but suicides. When investigating a hanging, the forensic expert should keep in mind that the manner of death in these cases is usually suicidal, sometimes accidental, and rarely homicidal. On the contrary, when a scene presents several characteristics of autoerotic deaths, this conclusion becomes highly probable, in spite of the method used. For example, if a man dies a nonnatural death in a secured house with a scene characterized by the presence of pornographic magazines, bondage, masochistic elements, and cross-dressing, this death is probably an autoerotic death as long as there is no clear element pointing toward a suicide. This conclusion would not be changed whatever is the autoerotic method that inadvertently caused death.

Case history: Bizarre death during autoerotic activity

Police officers were summoned to a residence to check on the welfare of a man who had not reported to work for 3 days. There was no response at his home. Officers were able to enter the premises via a closed and unlocked window. The interior of the home, which was unkempt, was putrid. The victim's two dogs had relieved themselves throughout the home. Nothing appeared to be removed or disturbed. When the officers checked the basement of the home, they discovered the dead 48-year-old, white, male victim. He was found burned and chained to a metal support column beneath an I beam. The deceased was chained in an upright position. He had Darby cuffs securing his feet, with a chain running from those Darby cuffs to his handcuffed hands and then to the top of the metal support column, where it was affixed to a padlock. Above his knees was another chain hooked with a clasp at his waist. A third chain wrapped around him and the pole and was secured with another small padlock (Figures 3.1 and 3.2).

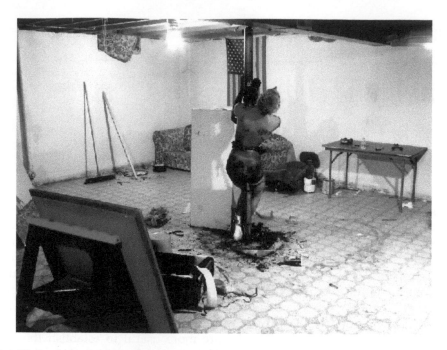

Figure 3.1 Victim bound with chains and burned. This was an equivocal death case since this event first appeared to be some sort of bizarre homicide. An examination of the crime scene and the victimology revealed this death was an autoerotic fatality. (Courtesy of Detective Sergeant Steve Gurka, Dearborn Heights, Michigan, Police Department; submitted from author Geberth's files.)

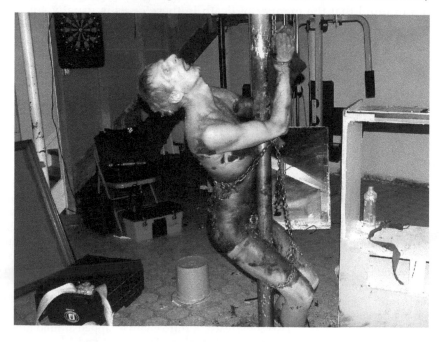

Figure 3.2 Close-up of victim chained to pole in basement. Note the chains around his waist and legs, highly suggestive of an assault. (Courtesy of Detective Sergeant Steve Gurka, Dearborn Heights, Michigan, Police Department; submitted from author Geberth's files.)

There were severe burns to the waist, chest, upper thighs, feet, and arms. A charred piece of cloth was wrapped around his penis, with the remnant of burned cloth at his feet. Soot was present in the mouth, lips, and teeth as well as around his nostrils.

The Darby cuffs on his feet did not have a key, and one could not be located in the area of the decedent. A handcuff key was also not present. The crime scene was searched, and the following items were discovered on the floor by the decedent's feet: some burnt cloth and ash, medical forceps, a glass "crack" pipe, electrical cord, a tow strap, a paper cup, a plastic bottle, and a cigarette lighter.

There was a dresser next to the victim's body. On the top of the dresser was a candle and melted candle wax and a set of keys for the padlocks; the dresser appeared to have been kicked back from its original position. The area in the basement around the victim contained the following items: a large mirror facing the deceased, a pair of pliers, a screwdriver, a hand drill, bolt cutters, cords, strapping material, and a weight bench (Figure 3.3).

The death was considered highly suspicious, so the body was transported along with the cuffs on his ankles and hands and the attached chains to the medical examiner's office. Toxicology indicated the presence of cocaine.

Interviews of family members and neighbors revealed that the deceased had been caught in the past by his mother while he was engaged in sexual gratification using handcuffs. This was important information in the final analysis of the manner of death.

The deceased basically kept to himself; he lived alone and did not date. On occasion, he would have some friends over from work to play poker. Interviews also revealed that the decedent had been introduced to crack by his older brother. The detectives had a forensic analysis of his computer done, which revealed over 300 JPEG images of preteen boys from Web sites.

The Darby cuffs had been ground out so that the victim could use the medical forceps instead of a key, which explained why there was no key for the cuffs (Figures 3.4 and 3.5). He was quite adept at binding and releasing himself from the cuffs using the

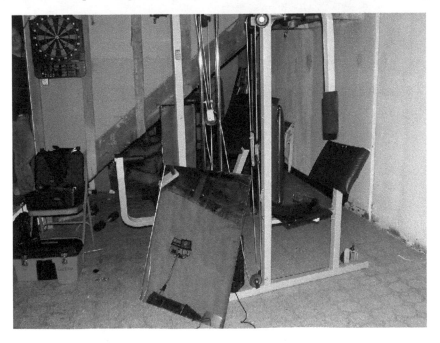

Figure 3.3 Mirror in the scene that the deceased was using to view himself. (Courtesy of Detective Sergeant Steve Gurka, Dearborn Heights, Michigan, Police Department; submitted from author Geberth's files.)

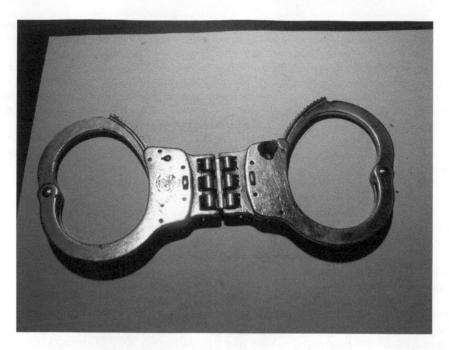

Figure 3.4 The Darby cuffs. (Courtesy of Detective Sergeant Steve Gurka, Dearborn Heights, Michigan, Police Department; submitted from author Geberth's files.)

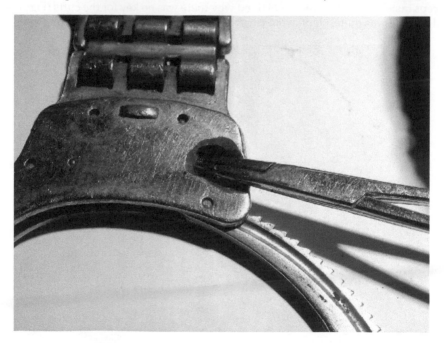

Figure 3.5 The victim had altered the cuff by grinding out the locking mechanism. He could use medical forceps instead of a key. (Courtesy of Detective Sergeant Steve Gurka, Dearborn Heights, Michigan, Police Department; submitted from author Geberth's files.)

forceps. At the time of the event, he was engaged in autoerotic cordophilia behavior for self-gratification.

The wood-topped dresser had originally been close to the victim so he could lean over and light his crack pipe. Apparently, the candle ignited his sweatshirt while he was under the influence of the crack. The victim had burned shirt material in one hand indicating his attempt to remove the burning shirt. The burning material fell onto his lap and ignited his shorts and socks. The manner of death was ruled accidental death due to autoerotic activity.

Having said that, the scene should never be interpreted in isolation. The other elements of the investigative triangle should be considered as well: the body (external examination or autopsy findings) and the history (see Chapter 2). If the autopsy reveals a natural cause of death, then despite all the scene characteristics, the death cannot be labeled autoerotic. If the history clearly reveals suicidal ideations, the possibility of suicidal intent should be further investigated; depending on the case, despite the presence of sexual features at the scene, the manner would be better ruled as suicidal or undetermined. The forensic expert should also keep in mind that the scene might have been staged. Sexual features might have been added to the scene in an effort to conceal a homicide. Or, oppositely, sexual features might have been removed from the scene by family members in an effort to preserve the deceased's reputation.

The forensic expert should also keep in mind that female autoerotic cases do not usually present with a florid scene. The sexuality of the female is different; their sexual fantasies are different and so is the scene in autoerotic death. This topic is further discussed in Chapter 7.

Case history: Female autoerotic death reported as a homicide

The victim was a 34-year-old schoolteacher who lived alone in an apartment a few blocks from her parents. She was single, heterosexual, and in good mental and physical health at the time of her death. On Saturday, she had spent the day with her parents, who were looking for a new home. They had dinner together that evening and had planned on meeting the next day. The father stated that he would call her the next day after church. On Sunday morning when the father was unable to make telephone contact with his daughter, he drove to her apartment and rang the bell several times and did not receive an answer. Her father then used a key, which his daughter had given to him to use in emergencies, and entered her apartment. Her father called out her name as he walked through the apartment and did not locate her. He then noticed the bathroom door was closed. He knocked and called out her name, but there was no response. When he opened the door, he found his daughter's seminude body hanging by a belt and a rope attached to the inside of the door (Figures 3.6 and 3.7). The hanging was a nontotal suspension with her feet on the floor. She was wearing a corset, and each of her breasts was bound with nautical ropes (Figure 3.8). Directly across from the victim was a full-length mirror that allowed her to observe herself in this position. The father called 911 to report what he believed to be a homicide. A search of the crime scene revealed evidence of prior autoerotic activity as well as additional nautical ropes in the bedroom closet. Investigation by detectives and consultation with the medical examiner resulted in a finding of accidental death due to asphyxia, and the case was classified as an autoerotic fatality.

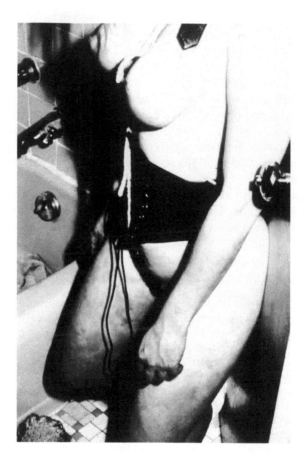

Figure 3.6 Female in partial suspension. This case was initially reported as a homicide. This photo shows the victim hanging from the back of her bathroom door. (Courtesy of Commander Tom Cronin, Chicago, Illinois, Police Department, retired; submitted from author Geberth's files.)

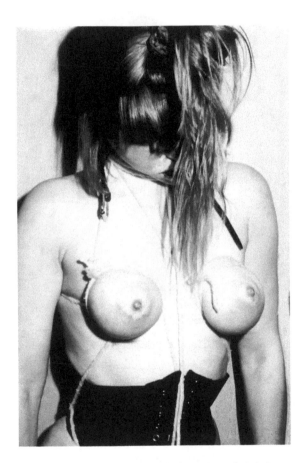

Figure 3.7 Her hair covered her face. There was a belt wrapped tightly around the victim's neck. (Courtesy of Commander Tom Cronin, Chicago, Illinois, Police Department, retired; submitted from author Geberth's files.)

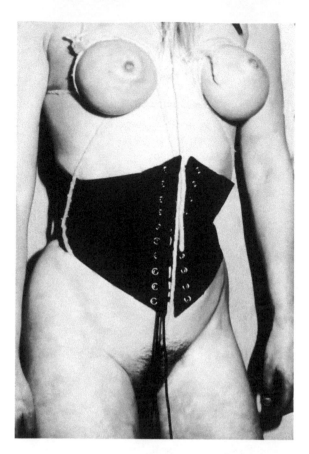

Figure 3.8 The ropes were wrapped tightly around each breast. One part of the rope extended through the labia and glutteal fold. The corset was also tightly secured around her abdomen. (Courtesy of Commander Tom Cronin, Chicago, Illinois, Police Department, retired; submitted from author Geberth's files.)

Common scene features

Fifteen scene characteristics can be encountered, in different combinations, at the death scenes of autoerotic deaths: nudity, exposure of the genitals, cross-dressing, evidence of masturbatory activity, foreign body insertion in the anus, lubricants, pornography, mirror, video recording, covering of the face (e.g., mask, duct tape), bondage of the genitals, other bondage, other masochistic behavior, protective padding in hanging, and evidence of repetitive behavior.

Nudity and exposure of the genitals

Commonly, the victim is found nude or with exposed genitals. This is an important clue to the possibility of an autoerotic death. However, not all dead bodies found nude or with exposed genitals are victims of autoerotic deaths. Not all victims of autoerotic deaths are found nude or with exposed genitals. It is important to realize that although a common aspect of a death scene in an autoerotic accident, genital exposure is not mandatory. This might seem surprising for some, but forensic experts should remind themselves that the direct stimulation of the genital organs is only one of the possible sources of sexual pleasure. For some individuals, the lack of oxygen in the central nervous system or the creation of fear and anguish in the context of masochism is the main source of their sexual pleasure, without the necessity to combine these sexual activities with masturbation (see Chapter 2).

Cross-dressing

The autoerotic practitioner is often found with some element of female dress: bra, panties, dresses, nightgown, nylon stockings, and high-heel shoes. The bra is often stuffed (with clothes, rice bags, plastic balls, etc.) to create breasts (Figures 3.9 and 3.10). Belts or ropes can be tied to create skin folds that resemble breasts. Wigs and makeup are other common props.

Apart from cross-dressing, other fetishism props can be encountered from time to time. It is impossible to address a complete list of possible fetishism elements since there is no limit to the human imagination and to the traditionally nonsexual objects or props that can elicit sexual excitation in some individuals. For example, at the time of death, one man was listening to the sounds of horses neighing.

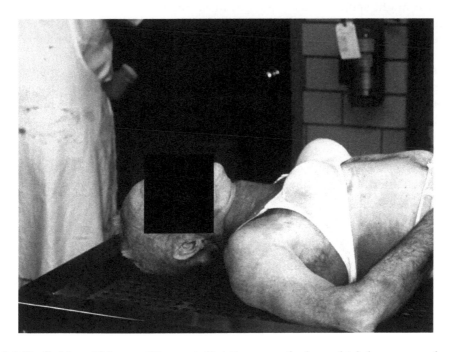

Figure 3.9 Stuffed bra. This practitioner stuffed the cups of a bra, which he wore under female clothing to give the impression of breasts. (Courtesy of Detective Lieutenant Raymond Krolak, Colonie, New York, Police Department, retired; submitted from author Geberth's files.)

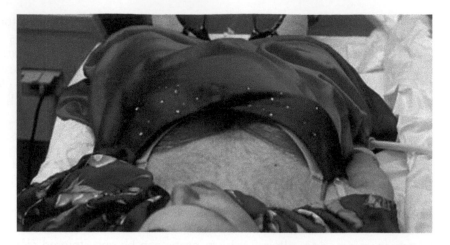

Figure 3.10 Breast prosthetics. This individual glued breast prosthetics onto his chest to resemble breasts. He wore women's undergarments and female clothing as he practiced autoeroticism. (Courtesy of Detective J. J. Mead, CSI, Columbus, Ohio, Police Department; submitted from author Geberth's files.)

Evidence of masturbatory activity

Evidence of masturbatory activity is sometimes found at the scene. However, contrary to what one might spontaneously assume, masturbation is not a mandatory feature of autoerotic practice. Quite the opposite—it is in fact an unusual feature. To be able to grasp the concept of autoerotic practice, again the forensic expert has to remember that sexual pleasure is obtainable not only through manipulation of the genital areas.

Evidence of masturbatory activity could be, for example, exposed genitals and paper tissues soiled with semen. The mere presence of semen on the penis or thighs, however, should not be considered to constitute evidence of masturbatory activity; it is known that postmortem "ejaculation" can occur.

It was thought previously that in case of hanging, ejaculation would occur during the agonal phase. In the study of filmed hangings performed by the Working Group on Human Asphyxia (see Chapter 4), this phenomenon was never documented. It is probable that the "ejaculation" observed in some cases was more a postmortem phenomenon, with discharge by gravity of a fluid.

Foreign body insertion in the anus

Various objects are found inserted in the anus: carrots, dildos, legs from chairs, and other items. The objects are sometimes still inserted in the anus at the scene, or sometimes they are found beside the body, soiled with feces (Figure 3.11).

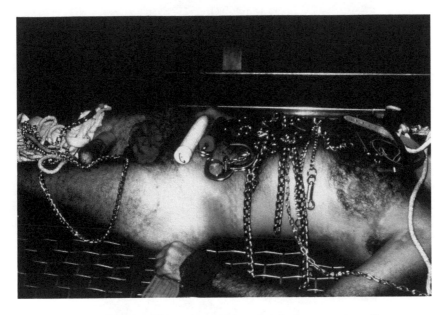

Figure 3.11 Objects in anal cavity. This autopsy photograph shows various items recovered from the scene of an autoerotic death. Note the fecal-stained dildo, which was removed from the victim's anal cavity during autopsy by the medical examiner. (From author Geberth's files.)

Lubricants

A jar or bottle of lubricant can be found in display at the scene of autoerotic death (Figure 3.12). Lubricant substances can also be noticed on the hand or genitals of the deceased, at the anus area, or on various objects used as sexual toys.

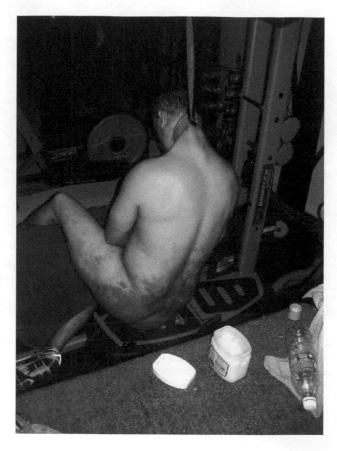

Figure 3.12 Lubricants recovered at an autoerotic death scene. (Courtesy of Detective Rich Kamholz, Rock County, Wisconsin, Sheriff's Department; submitted from author Geberth's files.)

Pornography

Pornographic material found in open view at the scene is a good clue to the possibility of an autoerotic death (Figure 3.13). To find pornographic magazines in the bedroom nightstand drawer or out of view in a storage area should not be overinterpreted. The exception to this is when the nature of the pornographic material found stored away is of a particular nature that gives an insight to the particular sexual fantasy of the individual: pornographic material related to autoerotic asphyxia, bondage, or masochism. Computers should also be searched for information on the types of Web sites visited by the decedent.

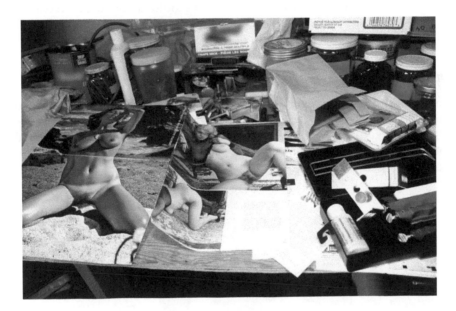

Figure 3.13 Pornography found in scene. (From author Geberth's files.)

Mirror and video recording

In the fantasy of the autoerotic practitioner, looking at the process can be an important part of the sexual excitement. In this context, mirrors are sometimes found displayed in a fashion that provides a good view of the "performance." Similarly, autoerotic practitioners sometimes take pictures or video record their practice.

Covering of the face, bondage of the genitals, other bondage, and other masochistic behavior

Masochistic elements are often encountered at the scene of autoerotic deaths. Bondage is quite common. The bondage can implicate nonsexual areas of the body, such as binding of the legs and arms. Binding of the genitals is also commonly seen, with bondage of the scrotum or penis.

    The face is sometimes covered by a blindfold, duct tape, or a mask. If the covering of the face is part of the autoerotic method per se, this should not be considered a further clue regarding the autoerotic nature of the death. For example, in suffocation by a plastic bag overhead, the covering of the face should not be counted as an autoerotic clue.

Protective padding in hanging

In hanging cases, the practitioner sometimes inserts a protection between his skin and the ligature (Figure 3.14). For this purpose, a towel, scarf, or piece of cloth is place between the neck and the ligature. This protective padding can be used either for personal comfort or to protect the skin from abrasions that otherwise could be noticed by family members, friends, coworkers, or clients.

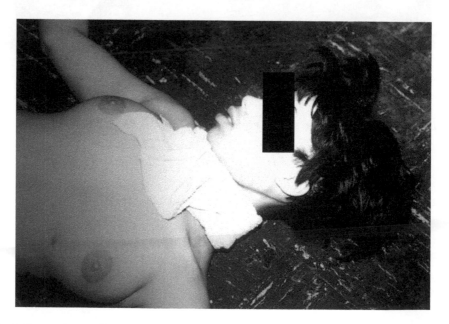

Figure 3.14 Protective padding. This victim was using a towel as padding to prevent any marking on her neck as she engaged in autoerotic activities. (Courtesy of Detectives Steven Little and Edward Dahlman, Columbus, Ohio, Police Department; submitted from author Geberth's files.)

This protective padding is not necessarily a sign of an autoerotic death. It is found at times in suicides, for the comfort of the victims.

Evidence of repetitive behavior

Although it is possible that an autoerotic death happens the first time that a victim practices a dangerous type of sexual solitary activity, there is generally a progression curve of risks taken by the practitioner, with death occurring after multiple previous increasingly dangerous activities. At the scene, there are sometimes signs of this repetitive behavior (Figure 3.15). For example, a ceiling beam can be found with several indentation marks from previous hangings. Or, a permanent hook can be found from which the victim was hanging in his basement. Multiple semen stains can be found on the walls and floor. Alternative bonding or cross-dressing options can be discovered in boxes or storage trunks.

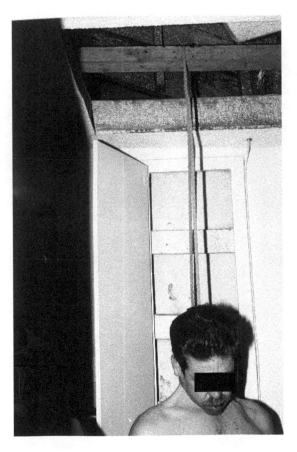

Figure 3.15 Evidence of prior autoerotic activity. This victim would hang nude in a closet in the bedroom of his house. He used a piece of 2 × 4 that spanned the access hole to an attic as the point of his suspension. The rope went around his neck and up over the 2 × 4 in the attic. The 2 × 4 had several indentations where the rope had rubbed in the past, indicating his prior autoerotic activities. (Courtesy of Detective Steve Mack, Huntington Beach, California, Police Department, retired; submitted from author Geberth's files.)

Case history: Typical autoerotic death—cross-dressed male

The victim was a 22-year-old male, who reportedly had been experimenting with asphyxial recreation for a number of years. The victim was hanging by the neck with an electrical cord secured to a 2 × 4 rafter above a ceiling tile, which had been removed to gain access (Figures 3.16 to 3.19). A printed scarf was between the ligature and the victim's neck. His body was discovered by his mother in the basement area of the family home.

At the time of his death, the victim was wearing a full-length lady's pink dress, and his hands were cuffed behind his back with handcuffs. He was wearing a brown woman's wig, women's shoes and underwear, and high-heel shoes. According to the victim's mother, her son had been wearing silky things and cross-dressing since he was 15 years of age. In 2009, he told his mother that he had been experimenting with autoerotic activities and had nearly lost his life on one occasion. This conversation took place after the autoerotic death of actor David Caradine, who was found hanging naked inside a closet at a Bangkok Hotel. The son maintained a room in the basement area where he kept his computer and women's clothing; detectives described the room as cluttered and filthy with a computer desk and computer. The mother had last seen her son at approximately

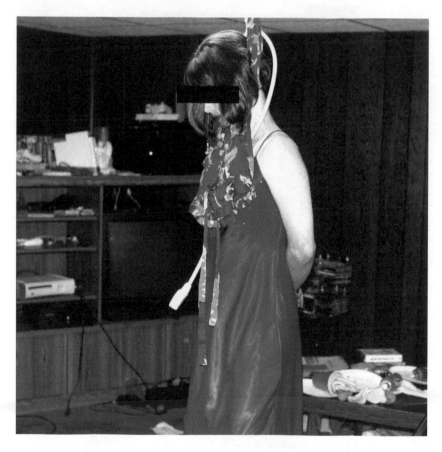

Figure 3.16 Full hang. This victim was discovered in a full hang suspended by the neck with an electrical cord secured to a rafter in the ceiling. He was wearing a full-length pink dress and high-heel shoes and had apparently slipped from the chair as he attempted to stop hanging. (Courtesy of Detective J. J. Mead, Columbus, Ohio, Police Department; submitted from author Geberth's files.)

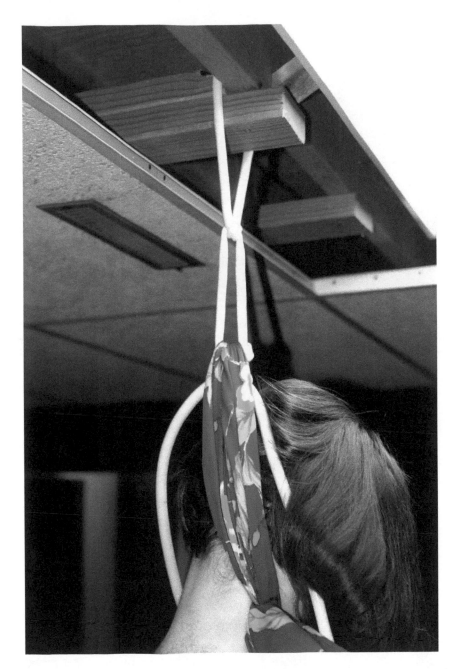

Figure 3.17 Ligature. The victim had removed a ceiling tile to reach the 2 × 4 rafter and secured an electrical cord noose around his neck with a scarf between his neck and the noose. (Courtesy of Detective J. J. Mead, Columbus, Ohio, Police Department; submitted from author Geberth's files.)

5:00 p.m. the previous evening and discovered him hanging at approximately 10:30 a.m. the next day.

While processing the crime scene, detectives noticed that the deceased had a computer-mounted camera (Figure 3.20) pointed in his direction. The detectives secured a search warrant for the computer, which was brought to their forensic office

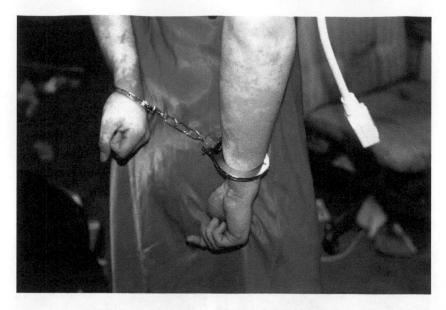

Figure 3.18 Handcuffs. The victim was able to cuff and uncuff himself according to the video tape viewed by detectives. (Courtesy of Detective J. J. Mead, Columbus, Ohio, Police Department; submitted from author Geberth's files.)

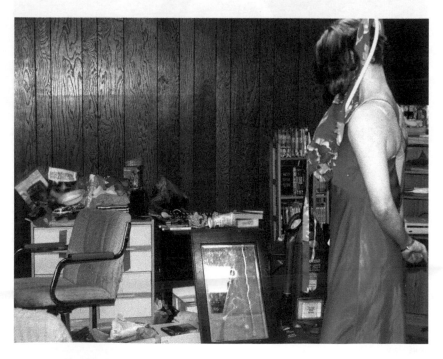

Figure 3.19 Mirror. Note the mirror in the crime scene; the victim could view himself as he engaged in autoerotic activity. (Courtesy of Detective J. J. Mead, Columbus, Ohio, Police Department; submitted from author Geberth's files.)

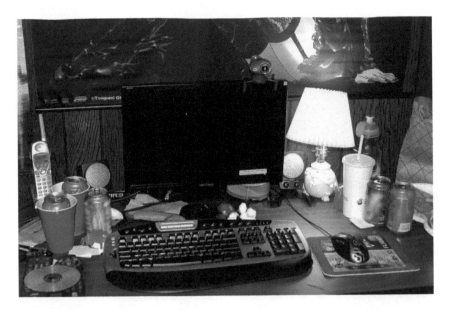

Figure 3.20 Computer-mounted camera. This was the camera that the deceased was using to record his activities, which aided detectives in reconstructing the entire events prior to and during his death. (Courtesy of Detective J. J. Mead, Columbus, Ohio, Police Department; submitted from author Geberth's files.)

for review. An examination of this computer revealed five videos dated the evening before his death with short clips of the deceased engaged in autoerotic activity. These clips were recorded at 5:06 p.m., 5:16 p.m., 5:21 p.m., and 5:24 p.m.

The final clip was made at 5:30 p.m. and recorded his death. This clip ran from 5:30 p.m. to 11:02 a.m. the next morning. The first four recordings showed the deceased wearing a short French maid's dress as he wore the brown wig and makeup. During these clips, the deceased was depicted cuffing and uncuffing himself while engaging in autoerotic activity. In the last clip, he was wearing the long pink dress with the high-heel shoes. As he attempted to get back up onto the chair, his long dress got caught on the high heels, and he slipped and hung to death.

Scene element forbidding ruling a death as autoerotic

The forensic expert needs to have good knowledge and understanding of the scene characteristics that constitute clues to the autoerotic nature of a death. Also very important, if not even more important, is to be aware that in order to be allowed to rule a death as autoerotic, there should be no clear elements indicating a suicide or homicide as the manner of death. The presence of a suicide letter at the scene forbids ruling the death as autoerotic unless it is strongly suspected or proven that the letter was placed at the scene in an attempt to conceal the sexual nature.

Case history: Autoerotic death—crime scene changed

Police were called to a home residence in connection with an unresponsive man. His wife stated that she and her children had gone to a high school football game earlier that evening and upon coming home could not find her husband. After looking in the garage they began going though the rooms in the house. The reporting witness discovered her

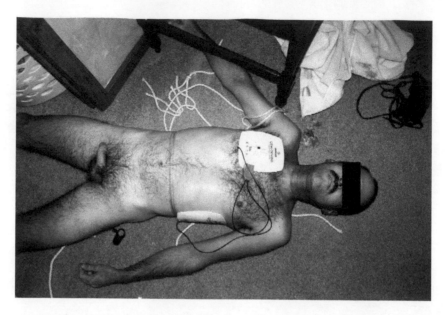

Figure 3.21 Body as found in scene. This was the position and condition of the body when the detectives first entered the crime scene. The paramedics had attempted resuscitation. There were numerous cut ropes around the body and obvious trauma to the victim's neck. (Courtesy of Detective Krystal Gibson, Criminal Investigations Bureau, Knox County, Tennessee Sheriff's Office submitted from author Geberth Files.)

husband hanging from some ropes attached to a hook in an upstairs bedroom closet. She stated that when she turned on the bedroom lights she at first thought that it was some kind of joke. She told the detectives that his feet were touching the floor and that he had some sort of black mask on his face. The woman yelled to her son to call 9-1-1. She told the police that she tried to get her husband down. However, she stated, "He had tied himself up really well." The woman then yelled to her son to bring her some scissors to cut her husband down. She and her son were then able to cut the victim down and they began CPR until the arrival of the paramedics (Figures 3.21 and 3.22).

The detectives took her statement and then conducted some preliminary observations of the scene. They observed the victim lying on his back in an upstairs spare bedroom and that his body was partially in the closet. They took note that the victim was totally nude. Directly in front of the victim's feet was a pair of black high-heel shoes. A pair of a scissors was lying next to the victim's left foot. A white towel was on the floor next to the victim's head. The victim had two distinct rope markings on or about his abdomen region as well as two distinct rope markings on his neck. A white vibrator was unplugged and laying on the bedroom floor. A part of the roping was also lying with the vibrator. (See Figures 3.23, 3.24, and 3.25.)

The lead detective, who had attended a Practical Homicide Investigation® course taught by one of the authors, immediately recognized the possibility that the death may be an autoerotic fatality and that the crime scene had been changed. She decided to personally re-interview the victim's wife in confidence regarding exactly what she had seen and what she had done prior to the arrival of emergency personnel. She asked a number of personal questions about their lifestyle and requested information about what sexual fantasies that she and her husband shared. She asked the woman whether or not she recognized the vibrator that was found in the closet. The wife stated that her husband liked to tie her up while she wore her one-piece bathing suit. She stated that the vibrator was hers and that she kept it in her bathroom in the same drawer as her curling iron and hair dryer. She was asked what size shoes she and her daughter wore

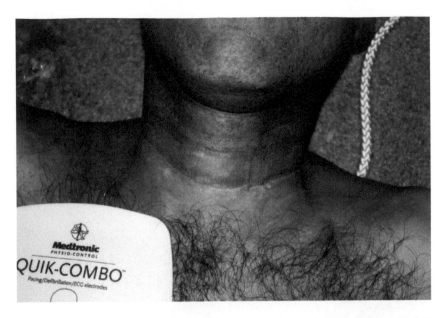

Figure 3.22 Ligature mark. Detectives noticed the prominent ligature mark around the victim's neck consistent with hanging. (Courtesy of Detective Krystal Gibson, Criminal Investigations Bureau, Knox County, Tennessee Sheriff's Office submitted from author Geberth Files.)

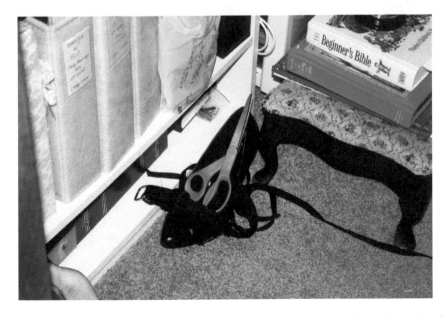

Figure 3.23 Scissors and high-heel shoe. Inside the closet detectives found a pair of scissors and the high-heel shoes, one of which is pictured herein. (Courtesy of Detective Krystal Gibson, Criminal Investigations Bureau, Knox County, Tennessee Sheriff's Office submitted from author Geberth Files.)

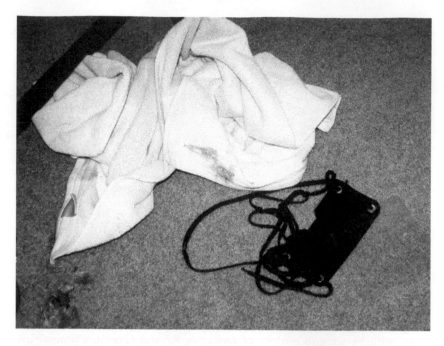

Figure 3.24 Black mask and towel. The wife stated that her husband had a black mask on when she found him. This mask was found on the floor along with a towel. (Courtesy of Detective Krystal Gibson, Criminal Investigations Bureau, Knox County, Tennessee Sheriff's Office submitted from author Geberth Files.)

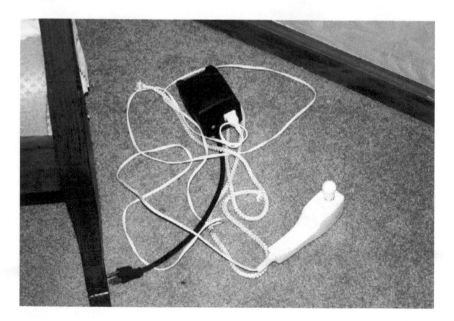

Figure 3.25 Vibrator. This vibrator, which was unplugged, was recovered in the scene. (Courtesy of Detective Krystal Gibson, Criminal Investigations Bureau, Knox County, Tennessee Sheriff's Office submitted from author Geberth Files.)

and she replied that they were 7 ½. She then remembered that when she first saw her husband hanging he had something black like a dog collar around his person and she removed it while trying to get him down.

The detectives then conducted a more thorough investigation around the bedroom, noting the victim's clothing and underwear tossed on the bed. They checked the black high-heel shoes and found that they fit the victim's feet and were a size 10. They located the black face mask in the closet and then found a woman's one-piece swimsuit and pantyhose stockings that had been wadded up and placed under a hat within a laundry basket in the closet where the victim had been found. When the detectives laid out the swimsuit and pantyhose on the floor they observed that the items had been cut up the side as if they had been removed from the victim (Figures 3.26 and 3.27). The investigators then noticed that a secured hook type apparatus had been attached with screws to a stud inside the closet above the closet door. The presence of this hook was highly suggestive that the victim had used this closet before to engage in autoerotic activity (Figure 3.28).

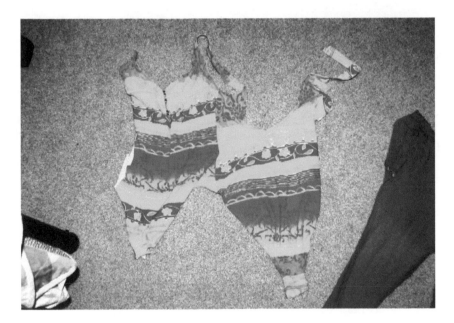

Figure 3.26 Bathing suit. These cut pieces of bathing suit were found wadded up and recovered from inside a laundry basket. (Courtesy of Detective Krystal Gibson, Criminal Investigations Bureau, Knox County, Tennessee Sheriff's Office submitted from author Geberth Files.)

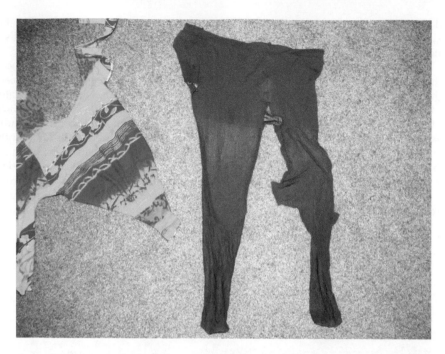

Figure 3.27 Cut pantyhose. These pantyhose had been cut from the victim's body. (Courtesy of Detective Krystal Gibson, Criminal Investigations Bureau, Knox County, Tennessee Sheriff's Office submitted from author Geberth Files.)

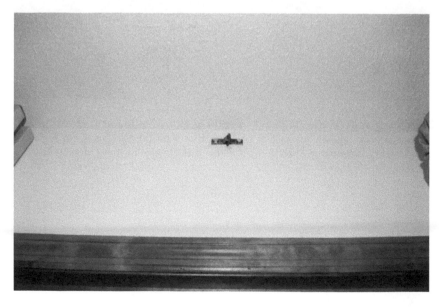

Figure 3.28 Hook apparatus. This hook had been screwed into a stud inside the closet door to allow the victim to hang inside the closet. (Courtesy of Detective Krystal Gibson, Criminal Investigations Bureau, Knox County, Tennessee Sheriff's Office submitted from author Geberth Files.)

The lead detective then re-interviewed the victim's wife regarding these items that were recovered by the detectives and she admitted that she had removed the bathing suit and pantyhose from her husband by cutting the garments off his body prior to the officer's arrival. She stated that she placed them in the laundry basket so they wouldn't be seen. She advised the detective that she was embarrassed for her husband and didn't know how to explain this event and that was why she removed these items. The investigators dutifully noted this in their report and there was no culpability on the part of the family.

Both of the authors agree that the actions of the wife under these circumstances were completely understandable. Some authors in literature have referred to these actions on the part of the family as "staging." However we disagree with that determination.

The "staging" of a scene is often done purposely by a perpetrator in order to mislead the police or to redirect the investigation in such a way that, for instance, a homicide appears to be a suicide. Staging, thus, is a conscious action of an offender, an attempt at a countermeasure; it does not refer to efforts taken by a surviving family member or other loved ones to cover or dress a victim in order to avoid embarrassment.

In this case the wife readily admitted why she had engaged in her actions. It was not to mislead the police nor thwart the investigation but to preserve the dignity of her husband.

This death was properly classified as asphyxia by hanging. The manner of death was ruled to be an accidental death, which occurred during a dangerous autoerotic practice.

A modern study of crime scene features in autoerotic death

The modern understanding of autoerotic death scene characteristics is still largely derived from the studies of Hazelwood et al. in the 1980s.[1,2] Despite the abundance of literature on autoerotic fatalities, there have been few studies that have reviewed and updated the description of the death scene. One of us recently conducted a study to fill this gap. The study was divided into two parts: a 25-year retrospective study of cases encountered in the province of Alberta (Canada) and a 30-year compilation of all published cases in the forensic literature.

For each case, the autoerotic method and the age of the victim were compiled, as well as the presence or not of these scene characteristics: nudity, exposure of the genitals, cross-dressing, evidence of masturbatory activity, foreign body insertion in the anus, lubricants, pornography, mirror, video recording, covering of the face (e.g., mask, duct tape), bondage of the genitals, other bondage, other masochistic behavior, protective padding in hanging, and evidence of repetitive behavior. Pornographic material was counted as present only if it was displayed at the scene (the presence of a pornographic magazine in a bedroom drawer was not counted); an exception to this was made for pornographic material that was directly related to autoerotic asphyxia, bondage, or masochism (in that case, the pornographic material was indicated as present even if hidden under the mattress or in a drawer). For the covering of the face, it was not indicated as present when the only covering of the face was part of the autoerotic method itself (e.g., in asphyxia by plastic bag). Lubricants were considered present if there was a jar or bottle displayed at the scene or if the substance was noticed on the hands or genitals. The mere presence of seminal discharge was not considered to constitute evidence of masturbatory activity.

Incidence of individual scene features

Of the 15 compiled characteristics, the most common feature of the death scene in an autoerotic fatality was the exposure of genitals (66%), followed by pornography (42%), nudity

Table 3.1 Incidence of Autoerotic Death Scene Features

Feature	Incidence (%)		
	Cases in Alberta	Cases from the literature	Overall
Nudity	45	39	41
Exposure of genitals	71	63	66
Cross-dressing	34	42	39
Evidence of masturbatory activity	8	16	13
Foreign body insertion in the anus	3	18	12
Pornography	50	37	42
Mirror	11	9	10
Video recording	5	0	2
Covering of the face	8	10	10
Bondage	50	30	37
Bondage of the genitals	26	15	19
Body bondage	34	25	29
Other masochistic behavior	11	13	12
Protective padding	11 (14% of hanging cases)	10 (25% of hanging cases)	10 (20% of hanging cases)
Evidence of repetitive behavior	8	7	8
Lubricants	13	9	10

(41%), cross-dressing (39%), and bondage (37%). Protective padding was present in 20% of the hanging cases. The other characteristics were present in 2% to 13% of scenes. The results for the cases in Alberta and from the literature were highly similar (Table 3.1).

This study indicated that none of the scene characteristics is always present. It also clearly demonstrated that the presence of protective padding is not mandatory to rule a hanging death as autoerotic. In fact, only one in five autoerotic hangings will present with protective padding. Mirror, video recording, and evidence of masturbatory activity are overall uncommon scene characteristics.

Number of scene features per case

On average, both cases compiled from the literature and cases from Alberta presented three characteristics per case (3.2 ± 1.5 for the compiled literature and 3.4 ± 1.6 for the Alberta cases). The most common combination of three features was exposed genitals, nudity, and pornography; this combination of three features was found in 19% of cases (15% of published cases and 26% of Alberta's cases).

In only 40% of cases were four or more features encountered at the scene (four or more scene features were found in 34% of published cases and 50% of Alberta's cases). The highest number of death scene elements compiled in a single case was seven for both the literature and Alberta's cases (with only one case from the literature and one case from Alberta presenting with seven characteristics).

In 11% of cases, only one scene feature was found at the scene (10% of published cases and 13% of Alberta's cases). Fewer than three scene characteristics were found in 33% of cases (33% of published cases and 34% of Alberta's cases).

This study demonstrated that forensic experts should not expect the presence of a long list of classic scene features in most cases. On average, only three scene features will be encountered. In certain cases, only one classic scene feature will be found, and after a full investigation of the case, including body examination and history review, this paucity of features at the scene does not necessarily advocate against ruling the death as autoerotic if the overall death investigation points toward that conclusion.

Comparison of scene features in relation to the autoerotic methods

The autoerotic methods were divided in three different groups: hangings (group 1), plastic bags and chemical substances (group 2), and atypical methods (group 3). The average number of death scene features was similar among the three groups (3.3 in hanging cases and 3.2 in both plastic bags or chemical substances and atypical methods).

The most common combination of three features in all three groups included exposed genitals and nudity. The third feature to complete the most common combination of three features differed depending on the autoerotic method: other bondage for hanging cases, pornography for plastic bag and chemical substances, and pornography and insertion of foreign body in the anus for the atypical methods.

By comparing the incidence of scene characteristics in these three groups of autoerotic methods, cross-dressing and the presence of a mirror were found significantly more commonly in hanging cases than in death with plastic bags or chemical substances and atypical methods. On the other hand, foreign body insertion in the anus and masochistic behavior were significantly more common in atypical autoerotic methods.

Comparison of scene features in relation to age group

The average number of scene characteristics differed in relation to the age group of the victim (Table 3.2). Death scenes in practitioners younger than 20 years of age generally presented with fewer scene features, with only two scene features on average.

Table 3.2 Average Number of Scene Features in Relation to Age Group

Age group	Average number of scene features
10–19	2.3 ± 1.3
20–29	3.8 ± 1.4
30–39	3.5 ± 1.6
40–49	2.9 ± 1.5
50–59	3.0 ± 1.5
60 and more	3.6 ± 1.1

Summary

In summary, death scene features are particularly important in establishing a death as autoerotic. The classic scene features of autoerotic deaths are nudity, exposure of the genitals, cross-dressing, evidence of masturbatory activity, foreign body insertion in the anus, lubricants, pornography, mirror, video recording, covering of the face (e.g., mask, duct tape), bondage of the genitals, other bondage, other masochistic behavior, protective padding in hanging, and evidence of repetitive behavior. Of these features, the most common were exposure of genitals (66%), pornography (42%), nudity (41%), cross-dressing (39%), and bondage (37%); the other characteristics were present in only 2% to 13% of cases.

On average, the forensic expert should expect three scene features per case. The most common combination of three features is exposed genitals, nudity, and pornography. In victims less than 20 years of age, this number is lower, at only two scene features on average. The presence of only one scene feature is enough if the rest of the death investigation points toward an autoerotic scene.

The forensic expert should keen in mind that the scene should never be interpreted without correlating with the autopsy finding and history review.

Scene characteristics: Checklist for the forensic expert

- Know that the death scene is the most important part in establishing a death as autoerotic.
- Never interpret the death scene in isolation; also consider the external examination or autopsy findings and the history.
- Know the 15 scene characteristics that can be found in autoerotic deaths: nudity, exposure of the genitals, cross-dressing, evidence of masturbatory activity, foreign body insertion in the anus, lubricants, pornography, mirror, video recording, covering of the face (e.g., mask, duct tape), bondage of the genitals, other bondage, other masochistic behavior, protective padding in hanging, and evidence of repetitive behavior.
- Be aware that exposed genitals or nudity is not mandatory for a diagnosis of autoerotic accident.
- Be aware that evidence of masturbatory activities is not mandatory for a diagnosis of autoerotic accident; on the contrary, it is a rare feature.
- Be aware that the mere presence of semen on the penis or thighs is not necessarily a sign of masturbation with ejaculation.
- Do not overinterpret the presence of stored pornographic material.
- Pay particular attention to pornographic material of a particular nature: material on autoerotic death, bondage, or masochism.
- Never rule a death as autoerotic if there are clear indications at the scene of a suicidal or homicidal manner of death.
- Know that the most common death scene features in autoerotic deaths are exposure of genitals (66%), pornography (42%), nudity (41%), cross-dressing (39%), and bondage (37%).
- Be aware that protective padding is present in only one of five autoerotic hangings.
- Know that mirror, video recording, and evidence of masturbatory activity are overall uncommon scene features.
- Expect on average only three scene features.
- Know that the most common combination of scene features is exposed genitals, nudity, and pornography.

- Be aware that the presence of only one classic scene feature is sufficient for ruling a death as autoerotic if that is the conclusion that seems the most appropriate after completing a full death investigation, including body examination and history review.
- For victims younger than 20 years of age, expect on average only two scene features.

References

1. Hazelwood RR, Burgess AW, Groth AN. Death during dangerous autoerotic practice. *Soc Sci Med* 1981;15E:129–133.
2. Hazelwood RR, Dietz PE, Burgess AW (eds.). *Autoerotic Fatalities*. Lexington, MA: Lexington Books, Heath, 1983.

chapter four

Typical methods of autoerotic deaths
Hanging*

Introduction

In a study reviewing all reported cases of autoerotic deaths over a 50-year span, it was concluded that typical methods of autoerotic activity leading to death were hangings and use of ligatures, plastic bags, chemical substances, and a mixture of these.[1] However, a standardization of the classification of asphyxia appeared in 2010,[2] and a strict application of definitions of ligature strangulation and hanging has an impact on this list of the most common methods. A revisitation of the typical method of autoerotic deaths, based on the new classification of asphyxia, was performed, and most cases previously called autoerotic ligature strangulation were now reclassified as hanging. Therefore, true ligature strangulation is an atypical method of autoerotic death. Typical methods of autoerotic deaths should now be considered to be hangings, followed at a distance by asphyxia by plastic bags and chemical substances.[3]

Indeed, hanging is by far the most common method of autoerotic activity leading to death, accounting for 40% to 80% of cases depending on the studies.[1,4–9] Since several cases that were previously called ligature strangulation would be reclassified now as hanging strangulation, it is probably more accurate to estimate the proportion of autoerotic hanging as close to 70% to 80% of autoerotic deaths.

Definitions of terms

Hanging is a type of strangulation, along with ligature strangulation and manual strangulation[2] (Table 4.1). Strangulation is defined as asphyxia by closure of the blood vessels or

Table 4.1 Definition of Terms

Term	Definition
Strangulation	Asphyxia by closure of the blood vessels or air passages of the neck as a result of external pressure on the neck
Hanging	A form of strangulation in which the pressure on the neck is applied by a constricting band tightened by the gravitational weight of the body or part of the body
Ligature strangulation	A form of strangulation in which the pressure on the neck is applied by a constricting band tightened by a force other than the body weight
Manual strangulation	A form of strangulation caused by an external pressure on the structures of the neck by hands, forearms, or other limbs

* This chapter was coauthored by Mark Benecke, PhD, and Lydia Benecke, MSc, both from International Forensic Research and Consulting.

air passages of the neck as a result of external pressure on the neck. If the pressure on the neck is applied by a constricting band tightened by the gravitational weight of the body or part of the body, the strangulation is classified as hanging. If the constricting band is tightened around the neck by a force other than the body weight, then the strangulation is called ligature strangulation.

Basic pathophysiology of hanging

When a hanging ligature is tightened around the neck, a compression of the neck structures ensues: jugular veins, carotid arteries, trachea, and vertebral arteries (Figure 4.1). The amount of pressure necessary to occlude the various neck structures is presented in Table 4.2. The jugular veins and carotid arteries are relatively superficial under the skin of the neck; therefore, a small amount of pressure is sufficient to obstruct the passage of blood in these vessels. The vertebral arteries are deeply located in the neck, on each side of the cervical vertebral column, and more pressure is required to close these vessels. However, these amounts of pressure, found in all forensic textbooks, were determined

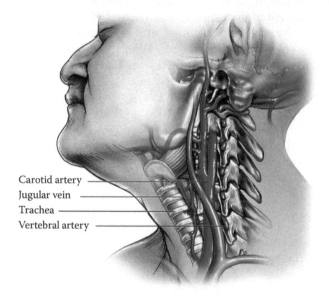

Carotid artery
Jugular vein
Trachea
Vertebral artery

Figure 4.1 Major blood vessels of the neck. Jugular veins, carotid arteries, trachea, and vertebral arteries. (Courtesy of Medical Legal Art. Illustration copyright 2010 Medical Legal Art, http://www.doereport.com.)

Table 4.2 Amount of Pressure to Occlude the Neck Structures

Structure	Amount of pressure required for occlusion
Jugular veins	2 kg (4.5 lb)
Carotid arteries	5 kg (11 lb)
Trachea	15 kg (33 lb)
Vertebral arteries	30 kg (66 lb)

in old cadaveric studies conducted at the end of the 19th and beginning of the 20th century.[10–12] Recent studies by the Working Group on Human Asphyxia, discussed further later in this chapter, have put in doubt the validity of these numbers.

Death in hanging has been traditionally attributed to three possible mechanisms[10]: closure of the blood vessels with lack of oxygen to the brain, compression of the airways, and vagal stimulation by pressure on the baroreceptors in the carotid sinuses and the carotid body.

Complete suspension versus incomplete suspension

The suspension of the body in a hanging can be complete or incomplete (Figure 4.2). In a hanging with complete suspension, the body is fully suspended by the neck, and the feet are dangling in the air above the ground. In incomplete suspension, on the other hand, parts of the body are touching the ground (Figures 4.3 to 4.5). Incomplete suspension hangings are subdivided into hanging standing with feet on the ground, kneeling, sitting, or lying. The proportion of the body weight applied on the ligature in these various positions has been studied by Khokhlov, and results are presented in Table 4.3.[13]

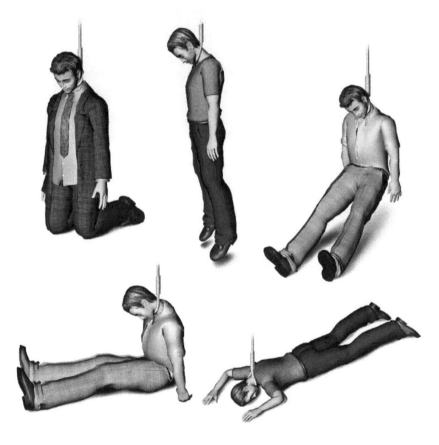

Figure 4.2 Hanging positions. (Courtesy of Medical Legal Art. Illustration copyright 2010 Medical Legal Art, http://www.doereport.com.)

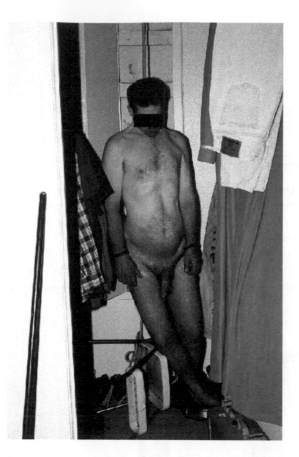

Figure 4.3 Autoerotic death: hanging in a standing position, feet on the ground. The completely nude male was hanging by a yellow rope, which was around his neck inside a clothes closet. The rope went around the victim's neck, up and over a 2 × 4 in the attic, and back down to the ladder in the closet where it was tied off. The victim had black leather wristbands around each wrist with a black leather strap connected to each wristband. The leather strap was wound though his crotch from the front of his body to the rear. The victim was hanging, but his feet were touching the floor with a slight bend in his knees. There was a two-step folding stool, which was tipped over to the right of his legs. (Courtesy of Retired Detective Steve Mack, Huntington Beach, California, Police Department. Reprinted with permission from V. J. Geberth, *Sex-Related Homicide and Death Investigation: Practical and Clinical Perspectives*, 2nd edition, CRC Press, Boca Raton, FL, 2010, p. 122.)

It might be surprising for some readers that death by hanging can occur without the body necessarily completely suspended in the air. However, it should be remembered that the weight of the head alone, on average around 10 pounds, is sufficient to close the jugular veins and even sometimes the carotid arteries. If only the jugular veins are compressed, the blood will not be able to drain away from the brain, and this vascular congestion will interfere with the supply of fresh oxygenated blood to the brain. If both the jugular veins and the carotid arteries are compressed, then the brain will lack both the blood drainage and the supply of fresh oxygenated blood by the internal carotid arteries, but the vertebral arteries will continue to supply blood.

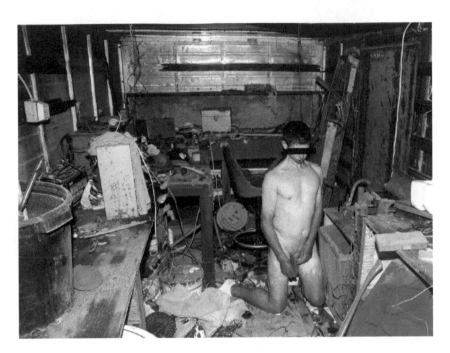

Figure 4.4 Autoerotic death: hanging in a kneeling position. This victim's body was found on the nursery and garden supply property by the victim's brother. The victim had made a secret room behind his workstation at the nursery that was not known by coworkers. It was a private work area where he could engage in this activity. There was sexual paraphernalia recovered in this room (whips, ball gag, etc.) and female lingerie, including panties and stockings and women's makeup. (Courtesy of Detective Scott Myers, Coral Springs, Florida, Police Department; submitted from author Geberth's files.)

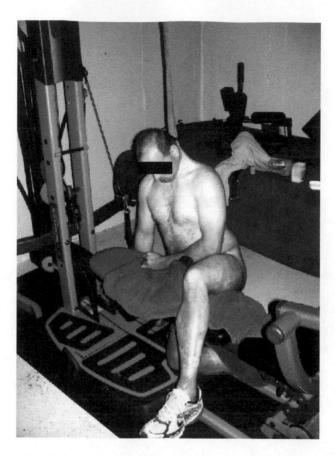

Figure 4.5 Autoerotic death: hanging in a sitting position. This victim was discovered sitting on a weight-lifting bench. The victim set a plastic-covered pipe wrench on the bench of the Bowflex® weight machine and then straddled the bench with the strap around his neck. He then began masturbating as he lowered his weight to tighten the strap and heighten his experience. The victim ejaculated and went unconscious, causing the strap to remain tight around his neck, which led to his death by asphyxiation. (Courtesy of Sheriff Robert Spoden, Rock County, Wisconsin, Sheriff's Department; submitted from author Geberth's files.)

Table 4.3 Proportion of the Body Weight Applied to the Hanging Ligature in Incomplete Hanging

Position of the incomplete hanging	Proportion of the body weight applied to the ligature
Standing, toes touching the ground	98%
Standing, feet flat on the ground	66%
Kneeling, buttocks down	74%
Kneeling, buttocks up	64%
Sitting, back suspended upright	18%
Sitting, back suspended backward	32%
Lying down, face down	18%
Lying down, face up	10%

Source: Data from Khokhlov, VD, *Forensic Sci Int*, 2001, 123, 172–177.

Variation of positions in autoerotic hangings

Autoerotic practitioners have been seen to use both complete and incomplete suspension in their practice. In complete suspension, they often use a nearby stool to start and end the body suspension (Figure 4.6). Less commonly, a ladder can be used (Figure 4.7). Incomplete suspension often involves a standing position with the mere flexing of the knees to get in and out of the partial body suspension. Autoerotic hangings in sitting and kneeling positions are also encountered and, rarely, even autoerotic hangings in a lying down position.

Two positions of autoerotic hangings deserve further comments. First, several victims kneel forward with a constricting band attached behind them to a bedpost or a doorknob. Because of the relative horizontality of the constricting band, these cases were previously classified as ligature strangulation by some authors. With a strict application of the definition of the standardized classification of asphyxia, these cases should be classified as

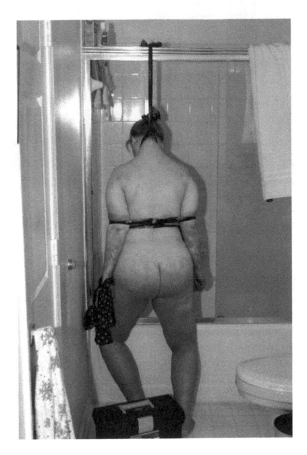

Figure 4.6 Toolbox step. The victim was in a semistanding position and completely nude with a piece of cloth with a slipknot in it around her neck. A search of the apartment revealed a number of sex toys and numerous items relating to sexual asphyxia, bondage, and autoerotic sexual activity. (Courtesy of Instructor–Coordinator John J. Wiggins, North Carolina Criminal Justice Academy, Department of Justice, State of North Carolina. Reprinted with permission from V. J. Geberth, *Sex-Related Homicide and Death Investigation: Practical and Clinical Perspectives*, 2nd edition, CRC Press, Boca Raton, FL, 2010, p. 160.)

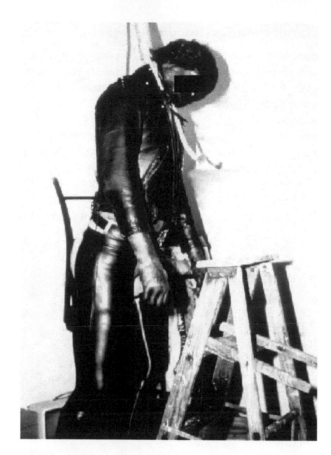

Figure 4.7 Typical autoerotic hanging. In this case, we see that the victim used a ladder to complete the suspension. (Reprinted with permission from V. J. Geberth, *Practical Homicide Investigation,* 4th edition, CRC Press, Taylor & Francis Group, Boca Raton, FL, 2006, p. 361.)

hangings. Indeed, despite the relative horizontality of the ligature (and this element is not relevant to the classification), the constricting band around the neck is tightened by the weight of the upper body.

Second, some victims are found lying down on their abdomens, with their ankles or feet tied to the neck (Figure 4.8). These cases also should not be called ligature strangulation. As a matter of fact, the asphyxia is caused by a constriction of the ligature around the neck by the weight of the legs; therefore, this is also a type of hanging. The fact that at some point there is a voluntarily movement done to create the asphyxia is irrelevant: The victim stepping from a stool to hang has also done a voluntarily movement, and no one will contest that this is nevertheless a hanging.

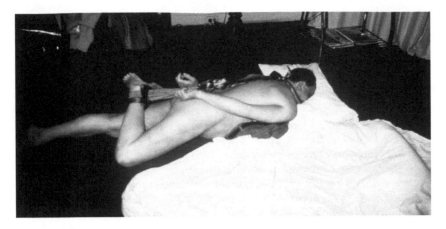

Figure 4.8 Autoerotic death: lying on floor. The victim was discovered in a New York City hotel room lying on the floor with his leg and hands bound in a hog-tied fashion. There was a ligature consisting of dress ties wrapped around his neck and joined with a bathrobe sash that was secured to his ankle, which he used to pull the ties tight around his neck to create hypoxia. At first, the authorities thought that they had a robbery homicide. However, the investigation indicated that the deceased had a history of engaging in autoerotic activities while on business trips. He had bound himself with neckties and towels from the hotel room. He had placed the sheets, pillows, and blanket from the bed on the floor to make himself more comfortable. He died from asphyxia. (From author Geberth's files.)

Scene investigation

The search of the crime scene is the most important phase of the investigation conducted at the scene. Decisions of the courts restricting admissibility of testimonial evidence have significantly increased the value of physical evidence in homicide investigations. Therefore, law enforcement personnel involved in the crime scene search must arrange for the proper and effective collection of evidence at the scene.

Physical evidence, which is often referred to as the "unimpeachable witness," cannot be clouded by a faulty memory, prejudice, poor eyesight, or a desire "not to get involved." However, before a forensic laboratory can effectively examine physical evidence, it must be recognized as evidence.

Practically speaking, anything and everything should be considered as evidence until proven differently. Unfortunately, quite frequently detectives have to return to a crime scene after receiving additional information that has revealed that some seemingly innocuous item was actually an important piece of evidence. That is why it is imperative to "hold on to" the crime scene as long as possible. Some item that did not seem significant on the first day of the investigation may suddenly take on the intrinsic value of gold.

In a hanging scene, particular care should be taken to describe and document the ligature with its loops and knots, as well as the type of suspension. In all deaths from hanging, if the victim is obviously dead, the body should not be cut down before proper photographic documentation and investigation of the scene have been conducted, and the ligature should not be cut from the body. First responders must be educated to the importance of leaving the body and scene intact if the victim is obviously dead, especially when dealing with microscopic evidence, which is subject to conditions and the environment as well as contamination during the crime scene response. There is no need to cut a body down from a suspension point or remove ligatures unless there is any chance of the person being alive.

Case history: Typical autoerotic deaths by hanging

A white, male in his late 40s, never married and living at home with his mother and sister, was found hanging in his basement workshop. He was wearing street clothing, which covered women's undergarments (a bra stuffed with padding, women's panties), women's boots, and leather gloves. A mask, which he had apparently been wearing, was found on the floor beneath him. He was hanging by a rope affixed to a hook in the ceiling (Figure 4.9). There was a Polaroid camera positioned on the workbench and a number of photographs of the deceased participating in this conduct. In his room, there were a number of pornographic magazines depicting female bondage, lesbian conduct, and sadomasochistic behavior. In addition to these commercial products, police discovered sadomasochistic drawings depicting the deceased dressed as a woman. In these drawings, this "woman" was observed with an erect penis threatening and abusing other women. There were also a number of these sexually explicit drawings of nude and seminude women urinating. These "fantasy drawings" were further illustrated with

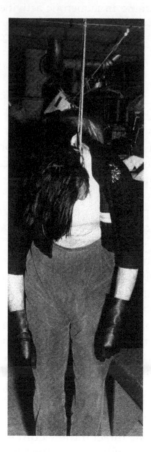

Figure 4.9 Autoerotic hanging. This victim was found hanging in the basement of the family home. He was wearing street clothing over women's undergarments. (From author Geberth's files.)

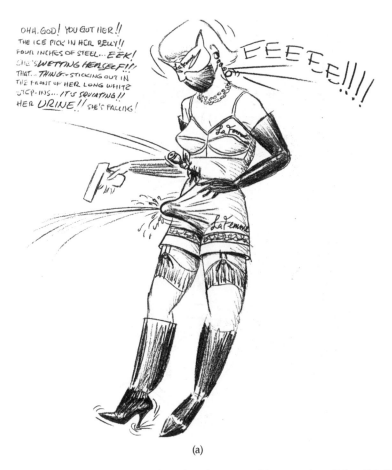

(a)

Figure 4.10 (a) and (b) Fantasy drawings found at the scene. (From author Geberth's files.)

words indicating that the deceased was actually verbalizing his sadomasochistic fantasies (Figures 4.10a and 4.10b). Also discovered were two legal-size sheets of paper listing approximately 200 pieces of woman's apparel and undergarments that the deceased had purchased. The victim had listed these items by number, description, price, and the name of the store from which the item was purchased. He then had a separate column, which indicated whether or not he had photographed himself in the item. This individual's total sex life was involved with solo sexual activities. His drawings further suggested paraphilias of transvestism, sadism, and masochism with fantasies of necrophilia and urophilia.[14] When advised of her husband's death, the ex-wife stated that this incident was probably due to his obsession with deviant sex. She told detectives that he was always "kinky," but toward the end of their marriage, "She just couldn't handle it." His fixation on bondage and pain during sex frightened her. The witness stated that she left him after finding women's attire in her house along with photographs of her husband dressed in sexy lingerie and in bondage. She stated that her husband took the pictures of her in lingerie found at the crime scene when they were married.

The case was properly classified as an autoerotic fatality based on the following considerations:

- The evidence of a physiological mechanism for obtaining or enhancing sexual arousal
- The evidence of solo sexual activity

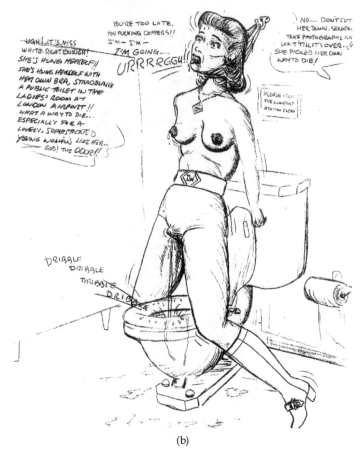

(b)

Figure 4.10 (continued) (a) and (b) Fantasy drawings found at the scene. (From author Geberth's files.)

- The evidence of sexual fantasy aids
- The evidence of prior dangerous autoerotic practice
- No apparent suicidal intentions
- The statements by his former wife relative to his kinky sex games as well as his past autoerotic practice
- The photographs of the victim engaging in autoeroticism
- The extensive collection of women's attire and lingerie

Case history: An equivocal death

Police were sent to a location to check on the welfare of a 36-year-old white male. When the officers arrived at the scene, they observed what appeared to be a female figure with blond hair hanging from a weight bench by a chain attached to the neck. On entry to the premises, they ascertained that the victim was in fact a male wearing a blond wig (Figures 4.11a and 4.11b).

The victim was discovered in the northwestern bedroom. He was dressed in female lingerie and wearing the blond wig, facial makeup, and nail polish on his fingernails. He was also wearing black fishnet hosiery, a black garter belt, a black corset, a black leather bra, and women's jewelry (Figure 4.12). In addition, he had a spiked leather collar, which was attached to a chain attached to the weight bench.

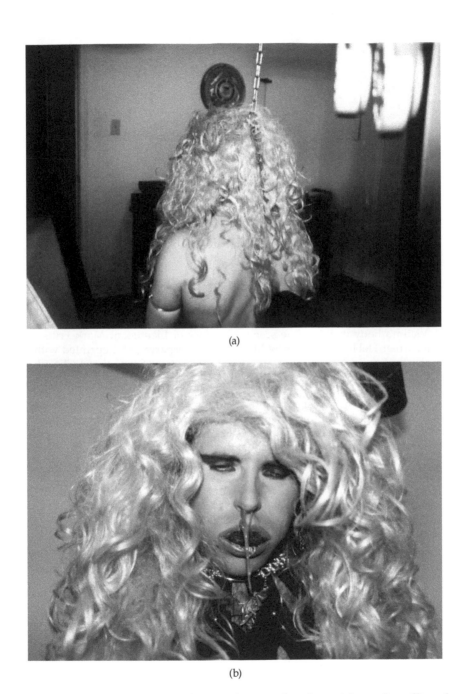

(a)

(b)

Figure 4.11 (a) and (b) Male autoerotic. This was the view that the arriving police officers had when they responded to the call. It appeared to be a woman victim. (Courtesy of Lieutenant Mark Fritts, retired, and Sergeant Pete Farmer Hobbs, retired, New Mexico Police Department. Reprinted with permission from V. J. Geberth, *Sex-Related Homicide and Death Investigation: Practical and Clinical Perspectives,* 2nd edition, CRC Press, Boca Raton, FL, 2010, pp. 164–167.)

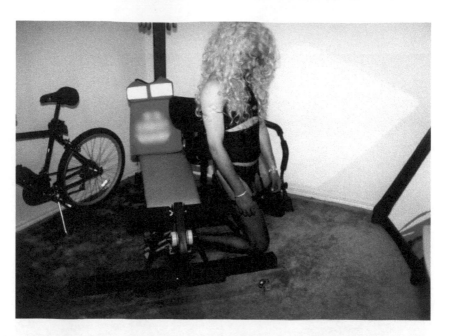

Figure 4.12 Victim's body in the crime scene. (Courtesy of Lieutenant Mark Fritts, retired, and Sergeant Pete Farmer Hobbs, retired, New Mexico Police Department. Reprinted with permission from V. J. Geberth, *Sex-Related Homicide and Death Investigation: Practical and Clinical Perspectives,* 2nd edition, CRC Press, Boca Raton, FL, 2010, pp. 164–167.)

A vanity mirror had been positioned in front of the subject, which provided an opportunity for the subject to view himself from his position in the room (Figure 4.13). There was evidence of sexual activity in the scene and a possible suggestion of another participant. However, an officer noted that the premises were secured, and there were no signs of forced entry.

During the search of the crime scene, detectives opened and looked into the victim's closet. They did not notice anything unusual at first. However, on closer examination they discovered numerous items of female attire secreted behind the regular clothing. The subject also had a number of pairs of women's panties in different sizes. He had women's high-heel shoes in a "large" size, pocketbooks, and nylon stockings.

In the adjoining room, the detectives observed that there was a black rubber dildo with fecal matter on it attached to the bedpost of the waterbed. Underneath the dildo was a hand towel and an open jar of petroleum jelly. There was a mirror placed on the floor with several Polaroid pictures. Some of these pictures were of a female dressed in lingerie, and glued onto these pictures was a simulation of a penis with bondage bands around the wrists. There were also other Polaroid pictures of the deceased wearing female attire and lingerie, involved in bondage scenes, and posing and simulating sexual activity. For instance, two Polaroids depicted the victim performing oral sex on a male partner. However, this turned out to be fabricated with a pair of stuffed jeans and a dildo. Apparently, the subject had been using the dildo as a sexual stimulus as he bent over and viewed the photographs, which were on the mirror.

Many sexual devices including various size dildos, were recovered in the house. There were different types of chains, restraint devices, handcuffs, nipple rings, and leather whips. The subject also had numerous sex magazines and pornographic tapes

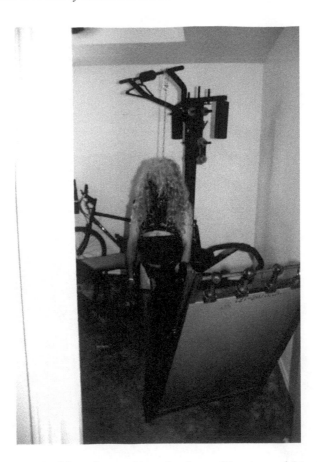

Figure 4.13 Male autoerotic. Note the positioned mirror. (Courtesy of Lieutenant Mark Fritts, retired, and Sergeant Pete Farmer Hobbs, retired, New Mexico Police Department. Reprinted with permission from V. J. Geberth, *Sex-Related Homicide and Death Investigation: Practical and Clinical Perspectives,* 2nd edition, CRC Press, Boca Raton, FL, 2010, pp. 164–167.)

as well as a nude anatomically correct Barbie® doll. In addition, police discovered a number of firearms hidden throughout the house in secret compartments. In the opinion of one of the authors whenever you have someone who is so thoroughly vested in pornography and this same person has access to a number of firearms, it is definitely a recipe for disaster.

Case history: Autoerotic death—sodomasochistic fantasy

A 35-year-old male expired during an autoerotic act involving sadomasochism. His fantasy focused on bondage. He had a black garbage bag over his head. His body was bound in several areas, with his feet tied together. His arms were bound behind his back with belts, which were attached to a metal hook. All of the bindings were interconnected and joined in a metal clasp that was attached to a rope with a loop knot, which was connected to a hook in the ceiling (Figures 4.14a–4.14c). As bizarre as this appears, the deceased was able to tie himself up in this fashion and reportedly had done this a number of times without injury.

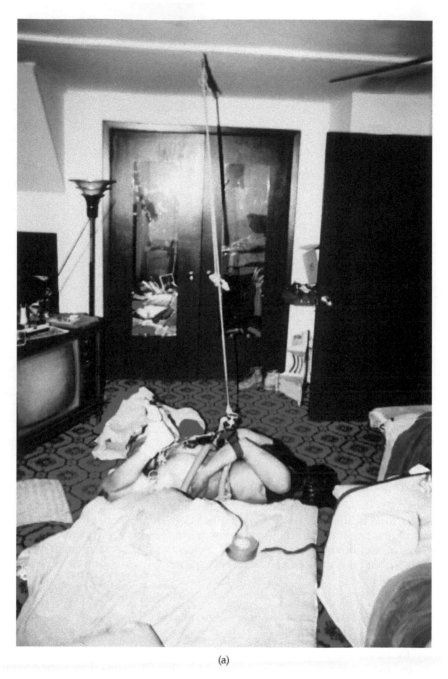

(a)

Figure 4.14 (a)–(c) Bondage. A 35-year-old male expired during an autoerotic act involving sado-masochism. His fantasy focused on bondage. All of the bindings were interconnected and joined in a metal clasp that was attached to a rope with a loop knot, which was connected to a hook in the ceiling (Courtesy of Sergeant David Vanderlpoeg, Village of Glenview, Illinois, Police Department. Reprinted with permission from V. J. Geberth, *Practical Homicide Investigation*, 4th edition, CRC Press, Taylor & Francis Group, Boca Raton, FL, 2006, p. 359.)

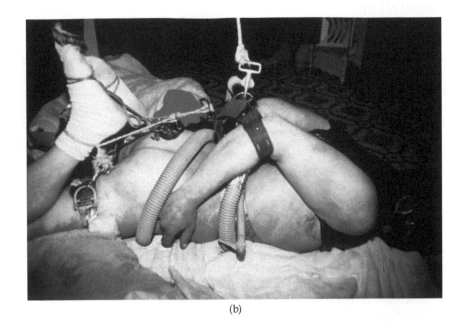

(b)

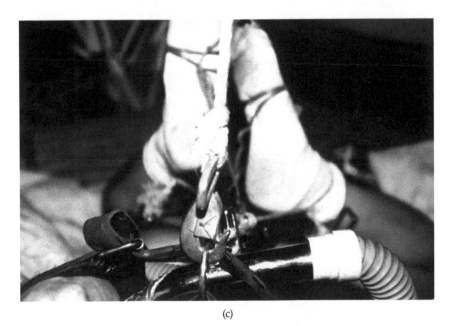

(c)

Figure 4.14 (continued) (a)–(c) Bondage. A 35-year-old male expired during an autoerotic act involving sadomasochism. His fantasy focused on bondage. All of the bindings were interconnected and joined in a metal clasp that was attached to a rope with a loop knot, which was connected to a hook in the ceiling (Courtesy of Sergeant David Vanderlpoeg, Village of Glenview, Illinois, Police Department. Reprinted with permission from V. J. Geberth, *Practical Homicide Investigation*, 4th edition, CRC Press, Taylor & Francis Group, Boca Raton, FL, 2006, p. 359.)

Body examination

Neck furrow

A ligature around the neck usually rubs or presses on the skin of the neck, producing an abrasion called a neck furrow (or ligature mark) (Figure 4.15). Depending on the type of ligature (rope, electrical cord, towel, necktie, belt, torn bedsheets, etc.), the clearness and pattern of the neck furrow will vary. Large and soft ligatures, such as towels or torn bed-sheets, generally create vaguely defined and faint neck furrows. In some cases, no recognizable marks are seen on the neck. On the other hand, thinner and stiffer ligatures, such as ropes or electric cords, generate better defined, well-demarcated neck furrows. The neck furrow sometimes presents a pattern corresponding to the ligature. For example, nylon ropes often leave behind a typical twisted pattern, and belts can be recognized by the neck furrow pattern with aligned holes and buckle imprint. A ligature made of textured textile can be recognized by a particular mirror-image impression in the neck furrow, for instance, waffle imprints corresponding to a bathrobe belt with similar texture.

Initially, the neck furrow has a pale yellow parchment-like appearance, with a congested rim. Over time, the neck furrow dries out and becomes more brownish.

If two loops are encircling the neck, two neck furrows can be found. If the skin is pinched between the loops, a hemorrhagic area can be created.

Usually, the neck furrow does not completely encircle the neck and is oriented diagonally to the neck. The neck furrow is deeper and better defined opposite the suspension point, with progressive fading toward the knot. The position of the knot or suspension point is most commonly at the back or the side of the neck. A knot or suspension point at the front of the neck is not impossible but is highly unusual.

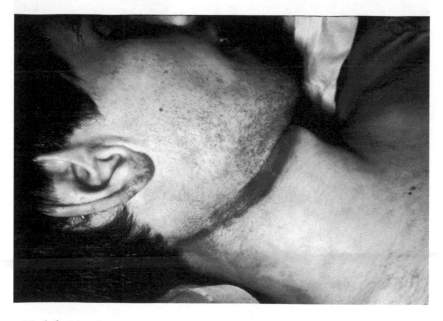

Figure 4.15 Neck furrow from ligature. (From author Geberth's files.)

Petechiae

Petechiae are pinpoint hemorrhages resulting from the rupture of small vessels (Figure 4.16). In hanging, mechanical obstruction of the venous return from the head causes an increase in intravascular pressure that induces overdistention of the thin-walled peripheral venules of the face. These overdistended vessels are then prone to rupture, creating petechiae. The venules located in areas that are low in connective tissue, such as the conjunctiva and sclera of the eyes, the skin of the upper eyelid, the forehead, behind the ears, and around the mouth, are more prone to rupture. Therefore, petechiae are most commonly observed in these areas.

Despite the fact that the presence of petechiae is considered one of the so-called classic signs of asphyxia, petechiae are not always present in hanging deaths. The incidence of petechiae in hanging varies greatly from one study to the next, from 23% to 69%.[15] This variation is easily explained: The incidence of petechiae is significantly higher in incomplete suspension compared to hangings with complete suspension; therefore, the general incidence of petechiae in different studies will vary significantly with the proportion of complete versus incomplete hangings in the series.[15]

Indeed, the incidence of petechiae in hanging with incomplete suspension is higher than in hanging with complete suspension. In incomplete hanging, the persistence of arterial blood supply in the absence of venous drainage generates high intravascular pressure in the face and head and a higher incidence of petechiae. On the contrary, it is believed that in complete suspension hangings the simultaneous blockage of both venous and arterial circulation creates stabilization without excess intravascular pressure. It is estimated that the incidence of petechiae in incomplete hangings reaches 40% to 60%, compared to 20% to 30% in incomplete hangings.[15]

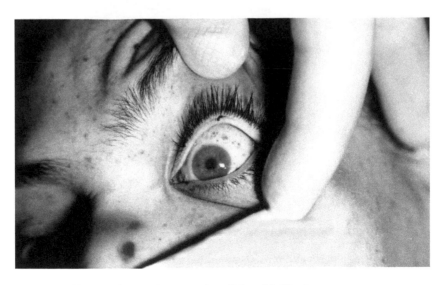

Figure 4.16 Petechial hemorrhages. (From author Geberth's files.)

Cyanosis, congestion, protrusion of the tongue

Cyanosis and congestion are other so-called classic signs of asphyxia that can be encountered in hangings. Cyanosis is a blue coloration of the skin and mucosa caused by excess deoxygenated blood. Congestion is an accumulation of blood by a diminution or obstruction of the venous drainage.

In hanging, the face can turn blue by excess of blood secondary to the blockage of the jugular veins. In most cases, however, the face stays pale since a simultaneous blockage of the arterial system impedes the excessive accumulation of blood in the face and head.

The ligature may press upward on the root of the tongue, causing it to protrude (Figure 4.17). The tip of the tongue, exposed to air outside the mouth, progressively dries out and blackens.

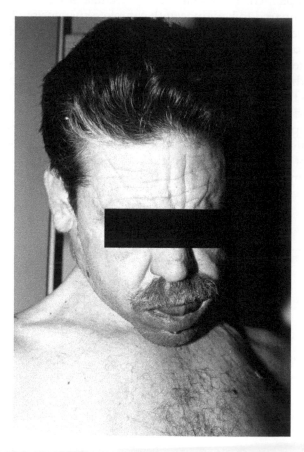

Figure 4.17 Tongue protruding. This is a classic example of the ligature pressing upward on the root of the tongue, causing a protrusion of the tongue. (Courtesy of Detective Steve Mack, Huntington Beach, California, Police Department, retired; submitted from author Geberth's files.)

Fractures of the neck structures

In suicidal and accidental hangings, the constriction of the neck may be associated with fractures of the hyoid bone or the thyroid cartilage (see anatomy in Figure 4.18). The incidence of such fractures varies greatly from one study to the next, from none to 77%.[16] By compiling all the available studies, a mean incidence of 37% was demonstrated.[16]

The incidence of fractures of the neck structures increases with age. As a matter of fact, neck structures become calcified and more brittle in middle and later life. Bony fusion of the greater horn and body of the hyoid bone is rare in an individual under 20 years old and increases with advancing age. The ossification of the thyroid cartilage also increases with the aging process, although there seems to be no direct correlation between the degree and frequency of ossification with increasing age.

A fracture of the cricoid cartilage, however, is virtually nonexistent in suicidal and accidental hangings.[16] By compiling all the literature, only one case of cricoid fracture was found in 2,700 cases.[16] Unfortunately, there are no details available on this isolated case of alleged suicidal hanging, and it could well be a missed homicide. It was recently proposed that since cricoid cartilage fractures are virtually nonexistent in suicidal and accidental hangings, whereas they are observed in 5% to 25% of homicidal strangulations, a fracture of the cricoid should be considered a potential pointer to homicide.[16] Of course, to conclude that a hanging is homicidal based solely on the presence of a fracture of the cricoid cartilage would be a mistake. In such a case, further police investigation should be recommended.

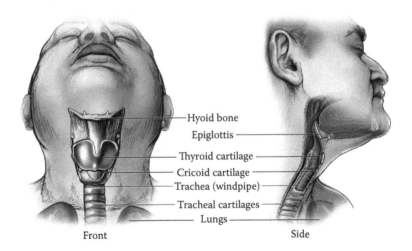

Front   Side

Figure 4.18 Anatomy of the neck structures. (Courtesy of Medical Legal Art. Illustration copyright 2010 Medical Legal Art, http://www.doereport.com.)

New data on the pathophysiology of hanging: The Working Group on Human Asphyxia

Until recently, the body of knowledge on the pathophysiology of hanging was still largely based on old writings from the end of the 19th century and beginning of the 20th.[10] This changed in 2006 with the creation of the Working Group on Human Asphyxia, an international research group that has a mission to regroup and analyze video recordings of human hangings. To date, 14 filmed hangings have been reviewed, including 9 autoerotic deaths.[17,18]

The agonic sequence in hanging

The agonic sequence in hanging is presented in Table 4.4. With time 0 representing the onset of hanging, victims rapidly lose consciousness in 8 to 18 s (average 10 ± 3 s). The loss of consciousness is closely followed by generalized tonic–clonic convulsions in 10 to 19 s (average 14 ± 3 s). The rapid loss of consciousness followed by generalized convulsions observed in filmed hangings is in keeping with results from an old and unusual study. In 1943, a research group in psychiatry carried out experiments on "volunteer" prisoners in the Stillwater State Prison in Minnesota.[19] A pneumatic cuff was inflated on the neck of 85 males to obstruct the jugular veins and carotid arteries while leaving the trachea unobstructed. Consciousness was lost in 5 to 11 s, followed by mild generalized tonic–clonic convulsions. The electrocardiographic changes were minimal, whereas the electro-encephalogram showed large, slow waves correlating with the loss of consciousness. The pressure of the pneumatic cuff was released after the loss of consciousness, and a full uncomplicated recovery was observed in all subjects within 1 to 2 min.

In the filmed hangings, a postural attitude called decerebrate rigidity followed the onset of convulsions. This postural attitude, observed at an average of 19 s (±5 s), is characterized by full extension of the upper and lower limbs, with extension of the hips and knees, adduction of the legs, internal rotation of the shoulders, extension of the elbows, hyperpronation of the distal parts of the upper limbs, with finger extension at the metacarpophalangeal joints and flexion at the interphalangeal joints (Figures 4.19 and 4.20).

Table 4.4 Agonal Sequence in Hanging

	Average time[a]
Loss of consciousness	10 ± 3 s
Convulsions	14 ± 3 s
Decerebrate rigidity	19 ± 5 s
Start of deep rhythmic abdominal respiratory movements	19 ± 5 s
Decorticate rigidity	38 ± 15 s
Loss of muscle tone	1 min 17 s ± 25 s
End of deep rhythmic abdominal respiratory movements	1 min 51 s ± 30 s
Last muscle movement	4 min 12 s ± 2 min 29 s

[a] From Sauvageau A, LaHarpe R, King D et al. *Am J Forensic Med Pathol* 2011;32(2):104–107.

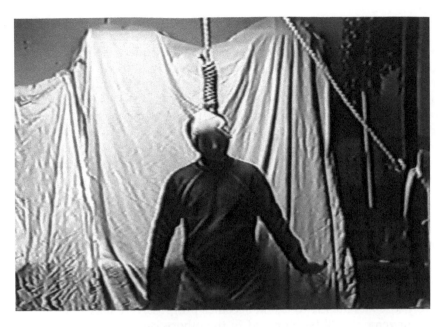

Figure 4.19 Decerebrate rigidity (still from a filmed hanging). (Reprinted with permission from V. J. Geberth, *Sex-Related Homicide and Death Investigation: Practical and Clinical Perspectives,* 2nd edition, CRC Press, Boca Raton, FL, 2010, p. 139.)

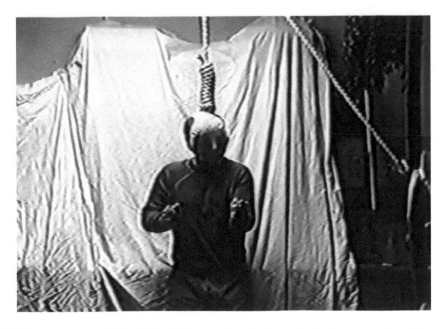

Figure 4.20 Decorticate rigidity. This still from a taped autoerotic death shows the victim in decorticate rigidity. (From author Geberth's files.)

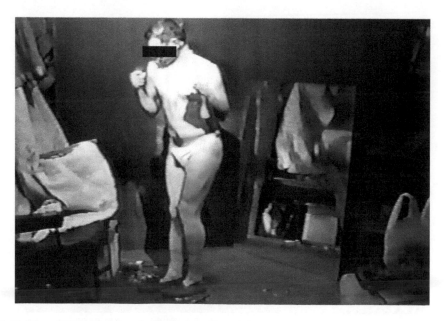

After the decerebrate rigidity, another postural attitude was observed, called decorticate rigidity. This postural attitude is characterized by marked extensor rigidity of the legs, identical to that observed in decerebrate rigidity but combined with rigidity of the flexors of the arms: The arms are flexed and bent on the chest, with the hands clenched into fists (Figures 4.21 and 4.22). In most victims, two or more phases of decorticate rigidity are observed, the first one occurring at approximately 38 s (±15 s).

Decerebrate rigidity indicates lesions at the midbrain level, whereas decorticate rigidity points toward cerebral cortex impairment. There is no clear explanation at this time why decerebrate rigidity generally precedes decorticate rigidity. Jugular veins and carotid arteries are more prone to occlusion by neck compression than are the more deeply located vertebral arteries. Considering that the midbrain is vascularized by tributaries of the vertebral arteries whereas the premotor areas of the cerebral cortex are vascularized by tributaries from the carotid, it could have been assumed that decorticate rigidity would appear first. However, this is not the case. Further research is necessary to achieve a better understanding of this phenomenon.

After slightly more than a minute of suspension (average 1 min 17 s ± 25 s), the body progressively loses its muscle tone and becomes progressively flaccid. From time to time, an isolated movement will be observed in the otherwise flaccid body. The last isolated body movement occurs between between 1 min 2 s and 7 min 35 s (average 4 min 12 s ± 2 min 29 s).

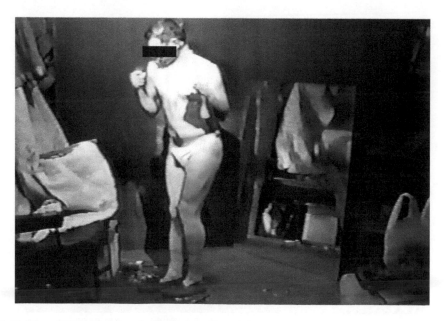

Figure 4.21 Decorticate rigidity (still from a filmed hanging). (Reprinted with permission from V. J. Geberth, *Sex-Related Homicide and Death Investigation: Practical and Clinical Perspectives,* 2nd edition, CRC Press, Boca Raton, FL, 2010, p. 140.)

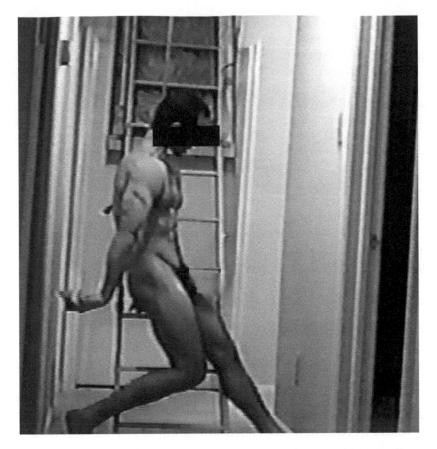

Figure 4.22 Decerebrate (still from a filmed hanging). Hands and arms hitting wall. (Courtesy of Detective sergeant Mark Reynolds, Harris County, Texas, Sheriff's Department; submitted from author Geberth's files.)

Respiratory responses to hanging

In the filmed hangings reviewed by the Working Group on Human Asphyxia, deep abdominal respiratory movements were clearly observed, with rhythmic rocking of the body by the contraction of the diaphragm.[17,18] These deep rhythmic abdominal respiratory movements started on average 19 s (±5 s) after the onset of hanging and stopped on average at 1 min 51 s (±30 s).

It is worth emphasizing that these respiratory movements not only are visualized but also are clearly audible, confirming the passage of air in the airways despite the hanging process. This observation strongly supports the notion that vascular occlusion is the major component of the pathophysiology of hanging. It should be pointed out that this last assertion is still controversial, and further studies are needed before concluding this old debate on the relative contribution of the three main possible mechanisms of death in hanging (occlusion of the airways, occlusion of the neck vessels, and vagal inhibition). Certain experts argue that the diaphragm and chest wall might appear to move as if the person is breathing, without air actually entering or exiting the lungs. The fact that abdominal "breathing movements" are seen does not necessarily mean that air exchange is occurring. This argument is easily disproved by the sounds of breathing heard on the hanging recordings. Some experts then argue that hearing breath sounds does not eliminate the possibility of significant airway obstruction. For example, many choking deaths with airway obstruction by food or foreign objects present with a partial pathway for air to move around the obstruction, yet these people still presumably died from airway obstruction. In hanging, if the trachea is compressed by a noose around the neck, there may be substantial narrowing of the lumen; despite that some air could still theoretically continue to pass by the area of compression, thus accounting for some degree of actual air passage. The mere fact that breath sounds can be heard does not definitely rule out respiratory obstruction as a mechanism of death in hanging. Ultimately, the studies of the Working Group on Human Asphyxia strongly support that tracheal occlusion is not complete in hangings, but it would be premature to totally exclude some implication of partial airway obstruction in the mechanism of death by hanging.

Study of filmed hangings casts doubt on the traditional conception of the pathophysiology of hanging

The study of filmed hangings by the Working Group on Human Asphyxia has cast doubt on the traditional conception of the pathophysiology of hanging.[17,18] The amount of pressure to close neck structures, as presented in Table 4.2 and found in all major forensic textbooks, makes no sense when put in parallel with the observation of filmed hangings.

For example, in the first case of the series of the Working Group, an adult male of 67.3 kg (148 lb) was found incompletely suspended in a standing position, feet on the ground. It was previously demonstrated that in a hanging in such a position, approximately 66% of the body weight is applied to constrict the ligature around the neck.[13] This percentage of the body weight corresponded in this case to about 44 kg (98 lb). Such a pressure around the neck is highly superior to the 15 kg (33 lb) required to completely occlude the trachea. It is nevertheless clearly audible in this filmed hanging that the victim presented deep rhythmic respiration, and that the trachea was not completely occluded. One possible explanation for this discrepancy between the traditional understanding of the pathophysiology of hanging and the observed reality might be that one important factor is often overlooked: the angle of the pressure on the structures of the neck. As a matter of fact, the weight necessary to occlude the various structures of the neck has been studied with pressure vectors applied perpendicularly to these structures. In real-life hanging, the pressure vectors are more diagonally oriented, with various angles to the neck depending on the position of the hanging.

Agonal responses to hanging in complete versus incomplete suspension

Until recently, it was generally thought in the forensic community that the time delay to the various elements of the agonal sequences in hanging would vary depending on the type of suspension. It was thought that complete suspension hanging would lead to death more rapidly than incomplete suspension hanging since the degree of neck obstruction is higher in complete suspension compared to incomplete suspension. These assumptions seemed reasonable and logical. The study of filmed hangings has nonetheless demonstrated otherwise.[17] Indeed, the agonal responses observed were strikingly similar in hanging with complete suspension and incomplete hanging standing, kneeling, and lying down.

Role of ischemic habituation on the agonal responses to hanging in autoerotic practitioners

Considering that autoerotic practitioners might develop over time a certain ischemic habituation, it is theoretically possible that these cases present a deceleration of the sequence. On the other hand, since they often play for a longer period with the hanging process before the final hanging, it could be argued that, on the contrary, their hanging sequence would be accelerated. Studies of filmed hangings have established that, overall, the time to the early responses to hanging (loss of consciousness, convulsions, decerebrate rigidity) seemed to be relatively similar between autoerotic hangings and suicidal hangings, with the exception of an accelerated start of deep rhythmic abdominal respiratory movements in autoerotic practitioners.[17] As for the late responses to hanging (decorticate rigidity, loss of muscle tone, end of deep rhythmic abdominal respiratory movements, last muscle movement), they seemed to be decelerated in autoerotic practitioners, but so far statistical analyses have confirmed this delay only for loss of muscle tone. Further research is needed to better define the effect of the ischemic habituation of autoerotic practitioners on the delay to the agonal sequences of hanging.

Role of ethanol in the agonal responses to hanging

In Canada, an expert witness recently stated that a victim intoxicated by ethanol would die more quickly from strangulation than a sober victim, alleging that ethanol is a respiratory depressant. This assertion was purely theoretical; there are no animal or human studies to sustain such an affirmation. The only available but limited study of this issue is a case of filmed hanging in a state of ethanol intoxication.[17] Based on this single case, ethanol intoxication does not seem to affect the timing of the agonal responses to hanging. Further research is needed to study the effect of ethanol and drugs on death by hanging.

Interpretation of bruises in hanging

External examinations of accidental autoerotic hanging victims occasionally reveal limb bruises. Such findings may raise suspicion of foul play or homicide. But, considering the postural attitudes of decerebrate and decorticate rigidity observed in the agonal sequences of hanging, such bruises are not surprising. In filmed hangings in restrained spaces such as hallways or bathrooms, the victim is often seen and heard to violently bang his hands and forearms backward on the wall during decerebrate rigidity and to strike his elbows while developing decorticate rigidity.

A comparative study of bruises in suicidal hangings and nonhanging homicidal strangulations established that the following pattern of bruises was usual and nonsuspicious in hanging: bruises on the posterior part of arms, bruises on the anterior part of legs, and bruises on either arms or legs but not both in a single case[20] (Figure 4.23). To find bruises on the anterior part of arms, on the posterior part of legs, or on both arms and legs is suspicious, and further investigation of the case, with full autopsy and scene review, should be considered.

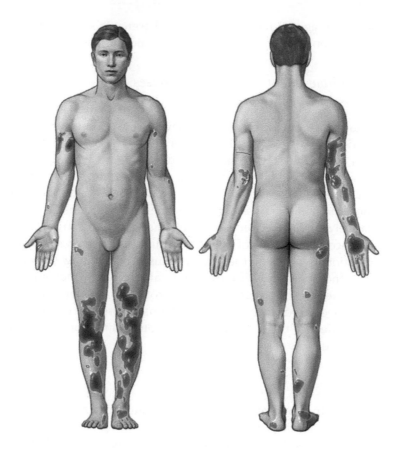

Figure 4.23 The usual pattern of bruises in hanging. (Courtesy of Medical Legal Art. Illustration copyright 2010 Medical Legal Art, http://www.doereport.com.)

Estimation of the time to die by hanging

It is widely said that the time to die by hanging is 3 to 5 min. Though this claim is deeply entrenched in the forensic community, an important article recently uncovered the lack of scientific evidence to sustain such an assertion.[21] No forensic study was ever conducted to point toward this estimate of 3 to 5 min to die. This dogmatic affirmation seems to be wrongly based on inappropriate extrapolation of three types of studies: a series of near-hanging victims in emergency medicine, studies of carotid endarterectomy, and animal physiopathological studies of brain ischemia.

A few studies have evaluated the outcomes of patients in unsuccessful hanging attempts (near hanging) by estimating the duration of the hanging based on the patient's estimate or from the family's report of when the patient was last seen.[21] Based on these studies, it is estimated that hanging of less than 5 min is survived by all patients, whereas no patient survives hanging of greater than 30 min. Such studies are strongly flawed: The duration of the hanging as estimated by the patients and family is certainly not precise, if not clearly erroneous. To estimate the duration of hanging from a patient's recollection does not make sense, particularly since it is known that the loss of consciousness occurs in seconds. As for the establishment of the duration of the hanging based on the time the patient was last seen, this is certainly also not a precise and valid measurement.

Retrospective studies of near-hanging victims are certainly useful to assess outcome predictors and complications of hangings but are not an appropriate method to estimate the time to die by hanging.[21]

Studies of carotid endarterectomy have clearly demonstrated that unilateral carotid clamping was tolerated without irreversible damage for more than 10 min in several patients.[21] Carotid endarterectomy is a surgical treatment of carotid artery stenosis that is effective, in selective patients, in preventing stoke. The goal of this surgical procedure is to remove the atherosclerotic plaque and to reconstruct the carotid artery. An inescapable risk of such a surgery is the clamping of the carotid artery, which puts the ipsilateral cerebral hemisphere at risk for ischemic change. Even though these studies have established that a unilateral clamping of the carotid artery is generally tolerated without irreversible damage for 10 min, very limited information about hanging can be drawn from these studies. Indeed, unilateral carotid clamping, contrary to hanging, is characterized by persistence of contralateral arterial carotid supply with natural arterial shunting through the circle of Willis and absence of obstruction of the venous return.

The fact that neurons undergo irreversible damage in 3 to 5 min of ischemia whereas myocardial cells can survive for 20 to 30 min is well known to all pathologists. Less known is that this timeline to neuron death is based on animal studies.[21] Despite the absence of human studies, thresholds for ischemic brain damage in rodents, pigs, cats, dogs, and nonhuman primates were extrapolated to humans. There is no doubt that animal in vivo models are useful and relevant to the study of mechanisms of ischemia. The generalization of animal data to humans is also certainly helpful for clinicians. However, it seems rather inappropriate and dangerous to apply these animal thresholds to forensic practice.

At this time, there is no study to support the generalized assumption that death in humans will occur in 3 to 5 min. Although this estimation is certainly precise and accurate enough for the needs of clinicians, it should not be considered strong enough to be used in forensic practice or in court.

Estimation of the time to irreversibility

The study of filmed strangulation by the Working Group on Human Asphyxia has revolutionized knowledge of the agonal sequence in such deaths; however, this study cannot provide the direct answer to the question of the time it takes to die by hanging. Indeed, on these videos it is impossible to evaluate the point at which the heart and brain death criteria are met. But, filmed hanging can be of help if we modify the question to the following: How long does it takes to reach an irreversible point? Said differently, at which point of the agonal sequences of hanging is death inevitable, even if the victim were to be unhooked and reanimation maneuvers were attempted?

To research this question, it was thought that nonlethal filmed hangings might be an interesting avenue of approach. By compiling data from nonlethal filmed hangings, the point at which the agonal sequence of hanging is still reversible could be documented, indirectly answering the question of the point of irreversibility.

A first study was conducted on three nonlethal autoerotic filmed hangings.[21] A 35-year-old Hispanic man was found to have filmed several of his autoerotic asphyxia sessions before his final lethal hanging. One of the filmed nonlethal hangings found at the scene was particularly interesting. In this short recording, the man hanged himself from the shower rod using a pair of pajama pants as a ligature. He lost consciousness, started convulsing 13 s after the onset of hanging, and presented a decerebrate rigidity at 20 s. The pants, which were not tied tightly enough, then detached from the shower rod, and the man fell to the ground, interrupting the hanging. The man quickly regained consciousness and seemed to present a full recovery without any noticeable symptoms.

This first study demonstrated that the first three early phases of responses to hanging are reversible: rapid loss of consciousness (10 ± 3 s), mild generalized convulsions (14 ± 3 s), and decerebrate rigidity (19 ± 5 s).

In the second study, published here for the first time, a movie from the sadomasochistic pornographic industry was obtained for research purposes, with consent from the women in the film, through a company producing and distributing sadomasochistic pornography. The authenticity of the movie was verified. In this video, a young volunteer woman is seen standing nude on a chair, with a loop of rope around her neck. She steps off the chair and hangs in complete suspension, feet off the ground (time 0). At 14 s, she tries to get back on the chair. She puts her right foot on the chair, but before she can put her left foot, she loses consciousness at 15 s. Her body falls backward, and her right foot pushes the chair away. Generalized tonic–clonic convulsions are observed starting at 16 s, rapidly followed by decorticate rigidity at 17 s and deep rhythmic abdominal respiratory movements at 18 s. A man standing in the same room pulls the rope down; the woman's feet are on the ground at 40 s, and she rests lying in a supine position at 44 s, at which time she is no longer hanging, and the constriction on her neck has ended. She presents decerebrate rigidity at 45 s and decorticate rigidity again at 50 s. The body relaxes to a neutral position at 1 min 16 s. She regains consciousness and gets up at 1 min 30 s.

Considering these two studies, it is now known that the initial responses to asphyxia by hanging are reversible: rapid loss of consciousness (10 ± 3 s), mild generalized convulsions (14 ± 3 s), and decerebrate rigidity (19 ± 5 s), onset of deep rhythmic abdominal respiratory movements (19 ± 5 s), and multiple phases of decorticate rigidity (38 ± 15 s). The point of irreversibility in hanging remains unknown at this time. Is it the loss of muscle tone (1 min 17 s ± 25 s), the end of the deep rhythmic abdominal respiratory movements (1 min 51 s ± 30 s), or the last isolated muscular movements (4 min 12 s ± 2 min 29 s)?

If one were to speculate concerning the time to die by hanging, the last isolated muscular movements might seem a reasonable irreversible point (4 min 12 s ± 2 min 29 s). Therefore, the belief that death happens in 3 to 5 min might not be wrong after all. However, this is speculation only, and there is no scientific evidence yet to support such assumption. Further research is needed. All forensic experts who come across a nonlethal filmed hanging are welcome to join the Working Group on Human Asphyxia; the data from these films will be added to the series, and the name of the contributors will appear in the list of authors.

At this time, the only honest and scientifically valid answer to how long it takes to suffer irreversible damage in hanging and other forms of strangulation remains that we unfortunately do not know. Series of nonlethal filmed hanging have demonstrated, however, that death by hanging is not a rapid type of death, and that neck constrictions of more than a minute are required.

Typical methods of autoerotic deaths: Checklist for the forensic expert

- List the typical autoerotic methods as hangings, plastic bags, and chemical substances.
- Do not list ligature strangulation as a common autoerotic method.
- Estimate the proportion of autoerotic hanging as approximately 70% to 80% of autoerotic deaths.

Basic knowledge in autoerotic hanging: Checklist for the forensic expert

- Define hanging as a form of strangulation in which the pressure on the neck is applied by a constricting band tightened by the gravitational weight of the body or part of the body.
- Be aware that hanging can occur with complete suspension or with incomplete suspension in a standing, kneeling, sitting, or lying position.
- Recognize as a hanging a victim found kneeling forward with a constricting band attached behind to a bedpost or doorknob.
- Recognize as a hanging a victim found lying face down with the ankles or feet tied to the neck.
- Pay particular attention at the scene to describe the ligature with its loops and knots and the suspension position of the body.
- Never cut down a hanging body that is obviously dead before proper photographic documentation.
- Never cut the ligature from the body in cases of obvious death.

Advanced knowledge in autoerotic hanging: Checklist for the forensic expert

- Know that a fracture of the cricoid cartilage in an apparent autoerotic hanging is a pointer to a potential homicide and recommend further police investigation.
- Know the agonic sequences in hanging: loss of consciousness in 8 to 18 s (average 10 s), followed by generalized tonic–clonic convulsions, decerebrate rigidity, decorticate rigidity, loss of muscle tone, and end of isolated muscle movements.
- Be aware that deep rhythmic abdominal respiratory movements persist in hangings.
- Be aware that bruises are a normal finding in hanging cases.
- Know the usual pattern of bruises in hanging: posterior part of arms, anterior part of legs, bruises on arms or legs but not both in a given case.
- Be cautious in the investigation of a hanging case with bruises of the anterior arms, on the posterior legs, or on both arms and legs.
- Do not claim as a fact that victims of hanging die in 3 to 5 min.

References

1. Sauvageau A, Racette S. Autoerotic deaths in the literature from 1954 to 2004: a review. *J Forensic Sci* 2006;51(1):140–146.
2. Sauvageau A, Boghossian E. Classification of asphyxia: the need for standardization. *J Forensic Sci* 2010;55(5):1259–1267.
3. Sauvageau A. A revisitation of the most common methods of autoerotic activity leading to death based on the new standardized classification of asphyxia. *J Forensic Sci* 2011; 56(1):261.
4. Sauvageau A. Autoerotic deaths: a 25-year retrospective epidemiological study. *Am J Forensic Med Pathol* 2012;33(2):143–146.
5. Blanchard R, Huscker SJ. Age, transvestism, bondage, and concurrent paraphilic activities in 117 fatal cases of autoerotic asphyxia. *Br J Psychiatry* 1991;159:371–377.
6. Breitmeier D, Mansorui F, Albrecht K, et al. Accidental autoerotic deaths between 1978 and 1997. Institute of Legal Medicine, Medical School Hannover. *Forensic Sci Int* 2003;137(1):41–4.
7. Behrendt N, Modvig J. The lethal paraphiliac syndrome—accidental autoerotic death in Denmark 1933–1990. *Am J Forensic Med Pathol* 1995;16(3):232–237.

8. Diamond M, Innala SM, Ernulf KE. Asphyxiophilia and autoerotic death. *Hawaii Med J* 1990;49(1):11–12, 14–16, 24.

9. Hazelwood RR, Burgess AW, Groth AN. Death during dangerous autoerotic practice. *Soc Sci Med* 1981;15E:129–133.

10. Clement R, Redpath M, Sauvageau A. Mechanism of death in hanging: a historical review of the evolution of pathophysiological hypotheses. *J Forensic Sci* 2010;55(5):1268–1271.

11. Brouardel P. *La Pendaison, la Strangulation, la Suffocation, la Submersion*. Paris: Bailliere, 1897.

12. Lacassagne A. *Précis de Médecine Légale*. Paris: Masson, 1906.

13. Khokhlov VD. Calculation of tension exerted on a ligature in incomplete hanging. *Forensic Sci Int* 2001;123:172–177.

14. Geberth VJ. Sexual asphyxia: the phenomenon of autoerotic fatalities. *Law Order* 1989;37(8):79–85.

15. Clément R, Guay JP, Redpath M, Sauvageau A. Petechiae in hanging: a retrospective study of contributing variables. *Am J Forensic Med Pathol* 2011;32(4):3728–382.

16. Godin A, Kremer C, Sauvageau A. Fracture of the cricoid as a potential pointer to homicide: a 6-year retrospective study of neck structures fractures in hanging victims. *Am J Forensic Med Pathol* 2012;33(1):4–7.

17. Sauvageau A, LaHarpe R, King D, Dowling G, Andrews S, Kelly S, Ambrosi C, Guay JP, Geberth VJ. The Working Group on Human Asphyxia. Agonal sequences in fourteen filmed hangings with comments on the role of the type of suspension, ischemic habituation and ethanol intoxication on the timing of agonal responses. *Am J Forensic Med Pathol* 2011;32(2):104–107.

18. Sauvageau A, LaHarpe R, Geberth VJ. Agonal sequences in eight filmed hangings: analysis of respiratory and movement responses to asphyxia by hanging. *J Forensic Sci* 2010;55(5):1278–1281.

19. Rossen R, Kabat H, Anderson JP. Acute arrest of cerebral circulation in man. *Arch Neurol Psychiatry* 1943;50:510–528.

20. Sauvageau A, Godin A, Desnoyers S, Kremer C. Six-year retrospective study of suicidal hangings: determination of the pattern of limb lesions induced by body responses to asphyxia by hanging. *J Forensic Sci* 2009; 54(5):1089–1092.

21. Sauvageau A, Ambrosi C, Kelly S. Autoerotic non-lethal filmed hangings: A case series and comments on the estimation of the time to irreversibility in hanging. *Am J Forensic Med Pathol* 2012;33(2):159–162.

chapter five

Typical methods of autoerotic deaths
Asphyxia by plastic bags and chemical substances*

Introduction

Hanging constitutes by far the most widely used method of autoerotic practice. In auto-erotic fatalities, 70% to 80% of deaths are attributed to hanging. Although less frequent, plastic bags and chemical substances are also commonly encountered methods of auto-erotic practice. These methods account for approximately 10% to 30% of autoerotic deaths.[1–5]

Definitions of terms

Subtypes of suffocation are asphyxia by plastic bags and asphyxia by chemical substances. Suffocation is a broad term encompassing different types of asphyxia, such as vitiated atmosphere and smothering, associated with deprivation of oxygen.[6] The new standard-ized classification of asphyxia recognizes three types of suffocation: smothering, choking, and confined space/entrapment/vitiated atmosphere (Table 5.1).[6] Smothering and chok-ing are both asphyxia by obstruction of the air passages. Depending on the level of the obstruction, the case will be classified as one entity or the other. The anatomical landmark that was chosen to distinguish both entities is the epiglottis: An obstruction of the air-ways above the epiglottis is called smothering, whereas an obstruction that extends below the epiglottis is classified as choking. The terms *suffocation in confined space, suffocation by entrapment*, and *suffocation in vitiated atmosphere* designate asphyxia caused by reduced oxy-gen in the air, by displacement of oxygen by other gases, or by gases that interfere chemi-cally with the oxygen uptake and utilization.

Table 5.1 Definition of Terms

Term	Definition
Suffocation	A broad term encompassing different types of asphyxia, such as vitiated atmosphere and smothering, associated with deprivation of oxygen
Smothering	Asphyxia by obstruction of the air passages above the epiglottis, including the nose, mouth, and pharynx
Choking	Asphyxia by obstruction of the air passages below the epiglottis
Confined space/ entrapment/vitiated atmosphere	Asphyxia in an inadequate atmosphere by reduction of oxygen, displacement of oxygen by other gases, or by gases causing chemical interference with the oxygen uptake and utilization

* This chapter was coauthored with Mark Benecke, PhD, and Lydia Benecke, MSc, both from International Forensic Research and Consulting.

Autoerotic deaths by plastic bags overhead constitute suffocation by smothering.[7] As for autoerotic deaths by chemical substances, in most cases the autoerotic practitioner used gases, such as nitrous oxide, propane, butane, ether, and aerosol glue, that caused suffocation by chemical asphyxia.[1]

Autoerotic deaths by smothering by plastic bags over the head

A plastic bag placed over the head leads to suffocation by mechanical occlusion of the external airways; the plastic bag will obstruct the passage of air through the nose and mouth. With filmy thin plastic, the bag clings to the face and, aided by condensation, sticks on the mouth and nose, directly obstructing the passage of air (Figure 5.1). With heavier, thicker plastic bags, such gluing of the plastic to the face is less common, and the bag usually needs to be secured at the neck to cause asphyxia; the victim exhales and inhales in a confined area without a supply of fresh oxygenated air. Progressively, there is a reduction in oxygen with an increase in carbon dioxide.

Autoerotic practitioners often secure the plastic bag at the neck by a loose ligature. In most cases, the ligature is loose and does not cause compression of the neck structures. In some cases, however, the ligature is tight enough to have caused ligature strangulation.

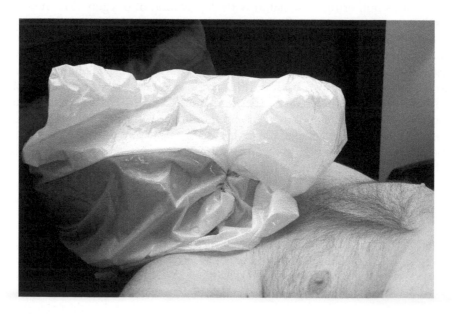

Figure 5.1 Plastic bag. Note that the plastic bag, which the victim had placed over his head to diminish oxygen intake, was sucked into the victim's mouth. (Courtesy of Investigator Perry Meyers, Lenexa, Kansas, Police Department; submitted from author Geberth's files.)

Scene investigation

In a scene of suffocation by plastic bag, particular care should be taken to describe and document the type of plastic bag; the position of the bag in relation to the head, mouth, and nose; and if the plastic bag is secured or not at the neck. If a ligature is present to enclose the bag, the type of ligature, with its loops and knots, should be described. Knots on the plastic bags should be documented as well. If the victim is obviously dead, the plastic bag should not be removed from the head before proper photographic documentation.

It is important to be aware that without proper scene information, the diagnosis of suffocation by smothering with a plastic bag over the head is most likely to be missed by the pathologist.

Autopsy findings

The autopsy findings in smothering by plastic bags over the head are nonspecific. Petechiae of the face, eyelids, conjunctiva, and mouth are usually not observed.

Pathophysiology of smothering

Two mechanisms have been proposed to account for these deaths.[8–11] First, the confined space created by the plastic bag could result, by rebreathing, in the progressive decrease of the oxygen concentration in the available inspired air. Second, the plastic bag could create a physical obstruction of the nose and mouth (smothering): The plastic bag becomes electrically charged and, with the associated condensation, adheres to the face. Some authors proposed, however, a third mechanism: The placement of a plastic bag on the face would stimulate the sympathetic nervous system, resulting in arrhythmias.[10–12] According to these authors, deaths by plastic bag over the head would be rapid, secondary to a cardio-inhibitory mechanism, and because of the rapidity of death by this mechanism, the other two proposed mechanisms of death would not have time to set in.[11,12] To further support the third mechanism as the most important, it was pointed out that most of these deaths do not present petechiae or other "classic signs of asphyxia," probably because of the rapidity of death.[11,12]

The agonal sequence in smothering is as follows: bradycardia (decreased heart rate), decrease in respiration to agonal gasps with eventual cessation of respiration, and slowing and finally flattening of the electroencephalogram.[8]

The literature to document the agonal sequences in smothering is scarce. The only documented case that we are aware of is the smothering of a 7-month-old female infant by her mother.[13] This was a classic case of Munchausen syndrome by proxy. The infant was investigated for recurrent cardiorespiratory arrest. According to the mother, the infant was presenting repetitive apneic spells. During these spells, the infant was found apneic, cyanotic, bradycardic, and unresponsive. After several minutes of resuscitation with oxygen ventilation and closed-chest cardiac massage, the infant would resume respirations. After several months of unsuccessful multidisciplinary investigation of the child, it was suggested that the mother might be inducing the apneic spells. The baby was monitored with electrocardiogram and electroencephalogram from a closed room, visually isolated from the technician. Two cameras were installed in the room: one wall-mounted camera in full view and one hidden camera recessed in the ceiling and covered by a grill. After several hours of video recording from the camera in full view, the camera was removed from the wall by electronics personnel, and the mother was told that the camera needed repair. Unaware of the hidden camera, the mother was seen to smother her child 2 h later by placing her left hand on the infant's right arm and the palm of her right hand on the baby's face. The hand smothering was maintained for 90 s, coinciding exactly with the apneic period. The heart rate started to decrease 30 s after the onset of the smothering. The electroencephalogram slowed and flattened after 90 s, becoming isoelectric for approximately 30 s.

There is no scientific study available at this time to establish the time to die by smothering in an adult. It is widely said that the time to die by asphyxia is 3 to 5 min. Although this claim is deep rooted in the forensic community, there is no scientific evidence to sustain such an assertion.[14] A discussion of this issue is presented in Chapter 4.

Pathophysiology of smothering: New data from the working group on human asphyxia

In a previously unpublished study of the Working Group on Human Asphyxia presented for the first time in this book, two nonlethal filmed asphyxias by plastic bag were analyzed. Despite the small number of cases, these films provide valuable insight into the pathophysiology of suffocation by placing a bag over the head.

The two cases of filmed nonlethal asphyxia by plastic bags were obtained, with consent from the two women involved, through a company producing and distributing sadomasochistic pornography. In these two videos, female volunteers were filmed in diverse sadomasochistic activities, including the application of a plastic bag over their heads. The authenticity of the films has been confirmed.

In the first video, the volunteer is tied sitting nude on a chair. There is bondage with ropes: Her legs are widely open, with the ankles tied on the back legs of the chair, her trunk is secured to the backrest, and her arms are tied at the back of the chair. The transparent plastic bag put over her head is only slightly bigger than her head, creating a relatively small confined space around the head. The plastic bag is moderately heavy and thick; it is not a thin, filmy plastic. The master* initially secures the bag at the neck by holding in tightly with his hands and then secured it with a metal collar over a protective textile padding (the collar seems tight enough to restrict the exchange of air but does not seem to be constricting the neck). The woman seems initially well and remains calm. Her mouth is slightly opened and she seems to be breathing without problems. The bag is seen moving inward and outward with each respiration. Over time, the bag starts to stick slightly on her nose and mouth. Forty seconds after the positioning of the bag over her head, the woman starts pushing the bag away with her tongue. This simple trick allows her to continue breathing without apparent difficulty. The adherence of the bag continues to build up, and even though she seems to push the bag harder and harder with her tongue, she starts having difficulties breathing; the bag is opened 3 min after having being placed over her head.

---

* The meaning of the term *master* is a top or dominant partner in a consensual BDSM (bondage, discipline, dominance/submission, sadomasochism) context. The master and the slave are both consensual persons in a consensual play scene. It is worth noticing that sexual offenders sometimes misuse the term, saying that they are the master but in a context that is no longer consensual.

In the second video, the volunteer is sitting nude on a chair, with bondage by tie wraps securing her ankles to the back legs of the chair, her trunk and upper arms to the backrest of the chair, and her wrists at her back. A tie wrap is put in her mouth, circling her head. A transparent plastic bag, similar to the one used in the previous case, is put over her head and secured at the neck with duct tape (the duct tape does not seem to be constricting the neck). The woman seems initially fine and breathes without apparent difficulty. Because of the tie wrap used as a gag, the woman has her mouth less open than in the first case, and this seems to lessen the amount of condensation produced. The presence of this gag also restricts her from using her tongue to push away the bag. At 1 min 45 s after the positioning of the bag overhead, the woman starts to present difficulties and exhales with increasing force to detach the bag from her face. The bag is opened at 2 min 4 s.

This study was the first to document the early agonal sequence in asphyxia by a plastic bag over the head. In both cases, there was no distress immediately following the placement of the bag over the head: The women were calm and breathing normally. The apparent distress was initiated when the bag started to stick on the nose and mouth. In the first case, the woman used her tongue to push the bag away, counteracting the adherence of the bag to her face. This allowed her to breathe relatively normally for up to 3 min. In the second case, a gag prevented the woman from using her tongue to detach the bag from her face. Despite her attempts to vigorously exhale to force the bag away, her distress occurred sooner, at 1 min 45 s, and the bag was opened at 2 min 4 s.

In these two cases, it is obvious that the mechanism involved in the distress was the physical obstruction of the nose and mouth by the plastic bag. In the event that the bags would not have been opened, it is almost certain that death would have occurred by smothering, that is, by the obstruction of the air passages above the epiglottis, including the nose, mouth, and pharynx. It is clearly seen in these films that the main problem was that, over time, the bag increasingly adhered to the face to a point that the method employed to counteract this adherence (pushing with the tongue or expiring with force) was finally overwhelmed.

It is difficult to evaluate if rebreathing in the confined space of the bag might have played a minor role in causing some muscular fatigue by hypoxia, with a secondary reduction in the efficiency of the method used to counteract the adherence of the bag. On reviewing carefully the videos on this aspect, it does not seem that the force of the methods used by the women was reduced over time. On the contrary, it seems that the women increased the force of their attempts over time to counteract the adherence of the bag, but this adherence increased in greater proportion. Therefore, at least in these two cases, rebreathing in a confined space did not seem to be an important mechanism.

As for the cardio inhibition following the stimulation of the sympathetic nervous system by the placement of a plastic bag on the face, there was no evidence of such a phenomenon in these two filmed cases. There was no early distress, and it does not seem that death would have occurred more rapidly than in other forms of asphyxia. On the contrary, it would seem based on these videos that the agonal sequence in asphyxia by overhead plastic bag is a slower sequence than the one observed in hanging and ligature strangulation.[15–17]

The time to die by asphyxia by plastic bag remains unknown at this time. This time would probably vary depending on the type of bag and the victim's characteristics. For example, the type of plastic and its thickness would probably interfere with the rapidity and the force of the adherence to the face. Furthermore, these videos demonstrated that the victim could use different methods to counteract the adherence of the bag, and these methods might change the rapidity of the sequence. It seems, however, that death is not particularly rapid and would probably take several minutes.

Autoerotic deaths by suffocation on chemical substances

Autoerotic practitioners often inhale aerosol propellants, chemicals, and gases to induce euphoric effects. Different props are commonly utilized to render the inhalation more efficient: masks, plastic bags, items of clothing. The most commonly used chemical compounds in the context of autoerotic practice are hydrocarbons, anesthetic compounds, and other chemical inhalants.

Case history: Autoerotic death by chemical substance

The victim was discovered by police after his friends had not heard from him for 5 days. The victim had been active in the gay leather bondage scene. The victim's body was in advanced decomposition when found. He was wearing a rubber gas mask with a canister attached; the canister contained an unknown chemical substance (Figures 5.2 and 5.3). When his body was discovered, he was clad in a leather thong, black elbow-length opera gloves, black support hose, and a silver-colored chain. The chain was wrapped around his waist and to his neck. Located beneath the crotch area was a tube of hand cream.

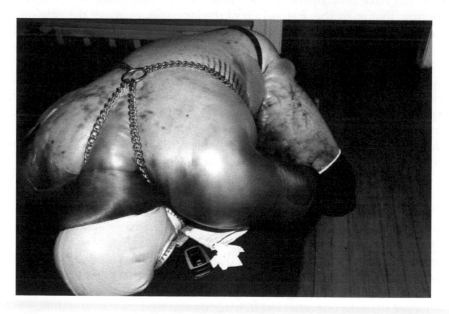

Figure 5.2 Chemical substance death. This victim was inhaling an unknown chemical substance while practicing autoerotic activities. (Courtesy Detective Mark Czworniak, Chicago, Illinois, Police Department. Reprinted with permission from V. J. Geberth, *Sex-Related Homicide and Death Investigation: Practical and Clinical Perspectives,* 2nd edition, Boca Raton, FL, 2010, p. 138.)

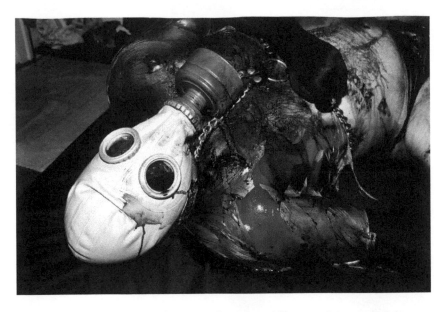

Figure 5.3 Victim's mask. Latex hood gas mask with a yellow canister containing an unknown chemical substance. The man was breathing through this mask and suffocated during an auto-erotic act. (Courtesy Detective Mark Czworniak, Chicago, Illinois, Police Department. Reprinted with permission from V. J. Geberth, *Sex-Related Homicide and Death Investigation: Practical and Clinical Perspectives,* 2nd edition, Boca Raton, FL, 2010, p. 138.)

Case history: Autoerotic death by refrigerant gas

The deceased was a 25-year-old male employed as a heating/ventilation mechanic. He had failed to report for work, and the police were requested to check on his welfare. Police officers forced entry into the residence and discovered the man lying facedown on his bed wearing his underwear in a bound position (Figure 5.4). He had bound himself, securing his legs, hips, and arms. The man was wearing a gas mask, which was attached to some tubing through which he was inhaling refrigerant gas from a canister below the bed (Figures 5.5 to 5.8). The gas was chlorodifluoromethane (Freon® 22), a colorless, near-odorless, nonflammable gas used in refrigeration. Inside the apartment, the police discovered numerous sexual devices and toys as well as a blow-up doll and "heavy leather" accessories. There was a video playing depicting a girl involved in sexual bondage. On the hot tub were numerous dildos and other sexual paraphernalia. The deceased had recently purchased hundreds of dollars worth of sexual devices online. He did not have a girlfriend and was basically a loner who spent a lot of time by himself at home.

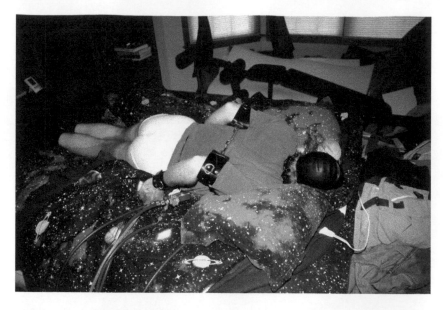

Figure 5.4 Victim in scene. This photo shows the victim lying facedown on his bed. He was wearing a gas mask, his arms were secured to his sides, and his hand was on the gas gauge of the refrigerant canister. (Courtesy of Detective Paul Koczwanski, Coventry, Rhode Island, Police Department; submitted from author Geberth's files.)

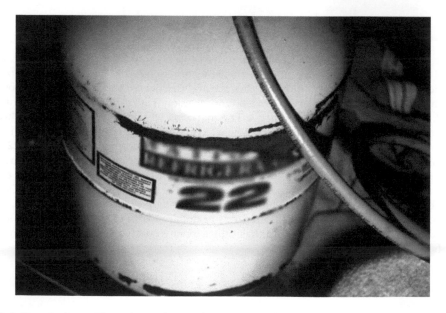

Figure 5.5 Gas canister. This photo shows the canister of refrigerant gas that the deceased was using to get "high" during his autoerotic event. (Courtesy of Detective Paul Koczwanski, Coventry, Rhode Island, Police Department; submitted from author Geberth's files.)

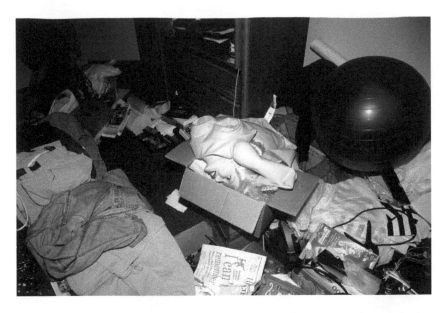

Figure 5.6 Paraphernalia. In the apartment, police discovered numerous sexual devices and toys as well as a blow-up doll and "heavy leather" accessories. (Courtesy of Detective Paul Koczwanski, Coventry, Rhode Island, Police Department; submitted from author Geberth's files.)

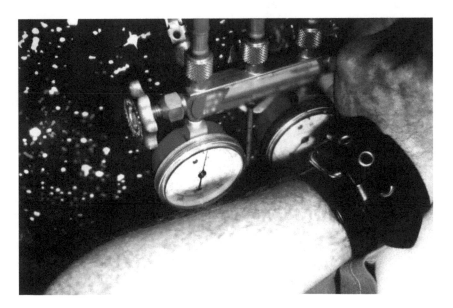

Figure 5.7 Gas gauge. This photo shows the man's hand on the gas gauge to control the flow of chlorodifluoromethane (Freon® 22) going into his mask. (Courtesy of Detective Paul Koczwanski, Coventry, Rhode Island, Police Department; submitted from author Geberth's files.)

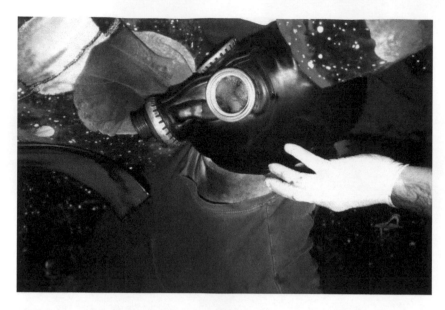

Figure 5.8 Gas mask. This photo shows the mask on the victim's face after it was disconnected from the gas supply hose. (Courtesy of Detective Paul Koczwanski, Coventry, Rhode Island, Police Department; submitted from author Geberth's files.)

Gaseous hydrocarbons

Hydrocarbons are organic compounds containing only carbon and hydrogen. They are the principal constituents of petroleum and natural gas. These chemical substances are found in fuels, lubricants, solvents, explosives, and industrial chemicals.

Hydrocarbons exist in different forms: gases (e.g., propane and butane), liquids (e.g., hexane and benzene), waxes (e.g., paraffin wax), and polymers (e.g., polystyrene). Autoerotic practitioners usually use gaseous hydrocarbons. Four gaseous hydrocarbons are known: propane, butane, ethane, and methane.

Propane is a gas that is heavier than air. It is also compressible to a liquid, and it is in this form that it is stored and bought (it is the type of gas used for common barbecue grills). Fuel gases sold as "propane" are mixtures of propane, isobutane, n-butane, methane, and ethane, with propane making up more than 90% of the chemical compound. Propane itself is a colorless and odorless gas, but an odoriferous agent (mercaptan) is added to the product for safety reasons, to simplify leak detection. Propane is nontoxic, but it can cause asphyxia through oxygen deprivation. The toxicity of propane is thought to be low, with probably high exposure concentrations in propane-associated deaths.[18] However, toxicity and mortality data in humans are limited.[18]

Butane is also a gas, compressible to a liquid. Natural gas is a mixture of gaseous hydrocarbons. The composition of natural gas varies widely, but it is usually formed primarily of methane; it can also contain a mixture of ethane, propane, butane, or pentane.

Anesthetic compounds

Inhalation of anesthetic gases such as nitrous oxide, ether, and chloroform is often encountered in autoerotic practice. These gases have euphoric and narcotic effects sought by practitioners. The use of intravenous anesthetics, although less common, has also been reported.

Inhalants: Glue, solvents, aerosols

A broad range of inhalants can be used by autoerotic practitioners to produce a high: the vapors of products such as airplane glue, Liquid Paper®, fingernail polish and remover, hair spray, deodorant, varnish, varnish remover, paint, enamel, lacquer, paint thinner, cigarette lighter fluid, charcoal lighter fluid, transmission fluid, gasoline, window cleaner, spot remover, dry-cleaning agents, and spray-on cooking lubricants. The solvent sometimes soaks a rag that is then inserted into the mouth to inhale the fumes; this practice is called *huffing*.

Numerous examples of inhalants are found in the literature. Isenschmid et al. reported the case of a 26-year-old man who was found dead at work.[19] The man, a security guard at a car dealership, was found dead in a conversion van, lying faceup on the floor between the seats. A plastic bag, containing a folded towel, was placed over the head and secured at the neck by a piece of panty hose. The body was clad in a nylon body stocking, with an opening at the crotch area and exposure of the genitals. Bondage elements were observed, with a leather belt at the waist, a piece of stocking material tied around the penis, and a long, thin piece of insulated wire loosely binding the wrists. A pressurized can of Fix-A-Flat tire repair was found near the body (this product contains a mixture of chlorodifluoromethane, tetrachloroethylene, and a trade secret compound). Toxicological analyses confirmed acute tetrachloroethylene intoxication. It seems that the decedent sprayed the chemical compound on the rag and then placed it inside the plastic bag.

In the work of Jones et al.,[20] the case of a 21-year-old man was described. The victim was discovered naked next to pornographic literature, with an overhead plastic bag containing aerosol glue spray.

Case history: Autoerotic death by plastic bag

Police were dispatched to an apartment complex at the request of the deceased's roommate, who advised them that he had discovered his roommate on his bed dead, inside his locked bedroom. The deceased was lying unclothed in his bed, with a white plastic "kitchen-type" trash bag over his head (Figure 5.9). The bag was semitransparent, and you could see that the victim was wearing his glasses under the bag. A portion of the plastic trash bag had been inhaled into the victim's mouth. A portable DVD player was on a nightstand next to the bed with the menu screen of a gay pornographic movie playing. A bottle of Astroglide® lubricant and a pink rubber/latex sexual aid were also located on the nightstand next to the bed. Lying on top of the bed, near the subject's feet, was a white plastic whipped topping dispenser. This dispenser utilizes nitrous oxide canisters as a propellant to dispense the topping (Figures 5.10 and 5.11). Near the subject's left leg were two boxes of EZ Whip nitrous oxide canisters. One of the boxes was opened and contained three unused canisters. The other box was still sealed and complete, containing a total of 24 canisters. Discovered scattered on the floor around the bed were 20 used nitrous oxide canisters. These used canisters, along with the one still contained in the dispenser and the 3 unused canisters still in the box, accounted for a complete box of 24 nitrous oxide canisters. Investigators learned from the deceased's' roommate that the victim regularly inhaled cartridges of nitrous oxide, referred to as "Whippits," by inserting the cartridges into a dispenser one after another and throwing them on the floor until he became high. He would reach a high about 15 min after inhaling half a box and then tilt his head back and start breathing heavily and be out of

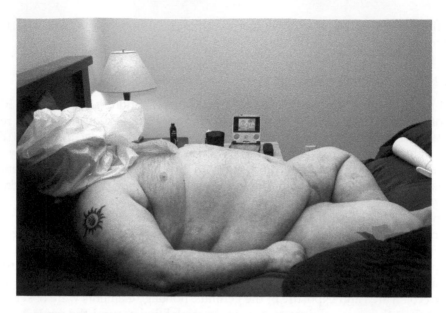

Figure 5.9 Body at scene. This was how the victim presented at the crime scene. (Courtesy of Investigator Perry Meyers, Lenexa, Kansas, Police Department; submitted from author Geberth's files.)

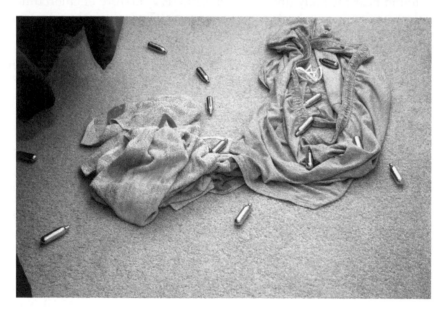

Figure 5.10 Nitrous oxide canisters. Victim's underwear is tossed onto the floor along with various empty nitrous oxide canisters, indicating heavy usage. (Courtesy of Investigator Perry Meyers, Lenexa, Kansas, Police Department; submitted from author Geberth's files.)

it for about 20 s. He would inhale a minimum of two boxes of Whippit on each occasion and would then pass out for about an hour and a half, with the whipped cream canister in his hand or next to his body. The deceased usually did this alone while watching pornography. The case was originally ruled a suicide by an inexperienced pathologist, who told the investigators, "I've never heard of them doing it that way." After educating the pathologist, he ultimately ruled that the death was accidental.

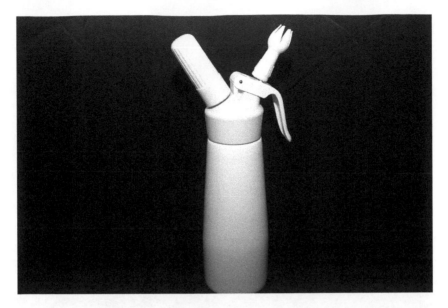

Figure 5.11 Whipped topping dispenser. Dispenser used to inhale the nitrous oxide found lying next to the deceased on the bed. (Courtesy of Investigator Perry Meyers, Lenexa, Kansas, Police Department; submitted from author Geberth's files.)

Other chemicals

Although less common, other categories of chemicals are sometimes encountered in the context of autoerotic asphyxia.

Case history: Autoerotic death—suffocation with ether

The 62-year-old white male was found lying on his back in the center of his bed in the second floor master suite; his legs were dangling off the side of the bed. The victim had a gag around his face, which was an Ace™ bandage wrap and a green washcloth held in place with duct tape. This covered the lower part of his mouth and chin, with his nose exposed.

The victim was completely naked except for a black leather strap with two wrist shackles on his wrists. His hands were cuffed with silver handcuffs with Ace™ bandages beneath the cuffs to prevent bruising (Figures 5.12 and 5.13). There was a plastic white zip tie connecting the black leather belt to the handcuffs. The key for the handcuffs was on the nightstand next to the victim. In the bathroom was a tan metal box containing dildos, leg restraints, hand restraints, lubricating jellies, and various other sexual devices. There was also a brown bottle containing a clear liquid, which examination revealed to be ether (Figure 5.14).

It was apparent that the victim had bound himself and placed the gag over his mouth. All of the towels and bandages were wrapped neatly around his face and wrists. The duct tape had been cut with scissors and carefully placed around the towels to hold them in place over his face.

Investigation revealed that the deceased would order Viagra® and ether over the Internet and had become sexually obsessed with autoerotic activity (Figure 5.15). His wife was away on a trip when this event occurred. The death was properly classified as an accidental death.

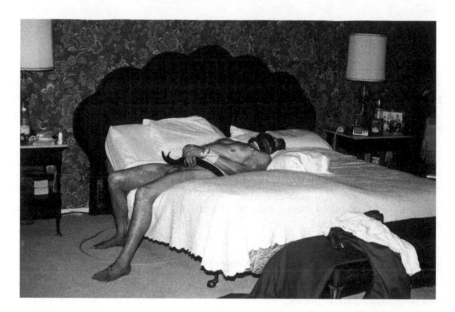

Figure 5.12 Body in crime scene. The body of the victim was discovered lying on his bed in bondage. (Courtesy of Detective Steve Mack, Huntington Beach, California, Police Department, retired; submitted from author Geberth's files.)

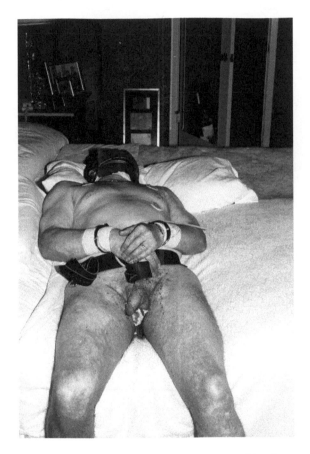

Figure 5.13 Close-up of victim's body. The victim had a gag around his face, with an Ace™ bandage wrap and a green washcloth soaked in ether held in place with duct tape. (Courtesy of Detective Steve Mack, Huntington Beach, California, Police Department, retired. Reprinted with permission from V. J. Geberth, *Sex-Related Homicide and Death Investigation: Practical and Clinical Perspectives*, 2nd edition, Boca Raton, FL, 2010, p. 154.)

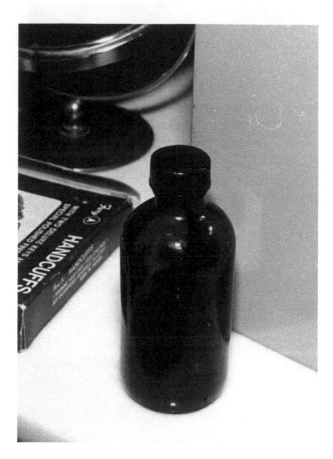

Figure 5.14 Bottle of ether. Recovered from crime scene. (Courtesy of Detective Steve Mack, Huntington Beach, California, Police Department, retired; submitted from author Geberth's files.)

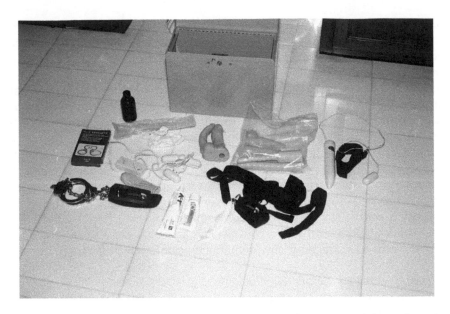

Figure 5.15 Paraphernalia. Sex toys and assorted paraphernalia recovered from the crime scene. (Courtesy of Detective Steve Mack, Huntington Beach, California, Police Department, retired; submitted from author Geberth's files.)

Scene investigation

Odors detected when entering the scene should be noted. The presence of a gas tank beside the body should be described, as well as the presence of a mask, plastic bag, or item of clothing on the face or head of the victim or beside the body.

Plastic bags, used in combination with chemical gases, can be submitted for toxicology analysis. To do so, bags should be put in an airtight can or glass jar (no plastic container) and refrigerated. Pressurized cans found at the scene should be seized and sent for toxicological analysis.

Scene investigators must be aware that some suffocating gases (e.g., helium) cannot be tested. Therefore, a proper scene investigation is mandatory to establish the cause of death.

Pathophysiology of propane-related deaths: New data from the Working Group on Human Asphyxia

In a previously unpublished study of the Working Group on Human Asphyxia presented for the first time in this book, a case of filmed propane-associated asphyxiation death was analyzed. This unusual case report is the first reported filmed event of this nature, and its analysis has important implications for toxicology, pathology, and scene interpretation.

A 44-year-old white man was found dead in his secured house, lying on the floor near an indoor propane heater. The man was wearing a mask connected by a plastic tube to the propane heater. The body was lying supine, both arms slightly overhead with flexed elbows.

A video-recording system had captured the lethal autoerotic event. The man is seen to install the mask over his head and to turn the gas on (time 0). He then lies on the floor and masturbates. Thirty-two seconds after the onset of gas flow, he stops masturbating and seems to have lost consciousness. At this point, the man is lying supine, his legs extended on the floor and his arms at his side with slightly flexed elbows. Deep rhythmic abdominal respiratory movements start at 33 s, and generalized tonic–clonic convulsions follow at 36 s. At 58 s, a postural attitude of marked extensor rigidity of the legs combined with rigidity of the flexors of the arms abruptly develops (decorticate rigidity). At 1 min 33 s, the deep rhythmic abdominal respiratory movements cease.

A second decorticate rigidity begins to develop slowly at 1 min 46 s and is sustained until 2 min 4 s. This second decorticate rigidity modifies the position of the arms at the scene. At the beginning of the decorticate rigidity, the arms rest on the side of the body, with the palms of the hands facing downward. During the course of the decorticate rigidity, the forearms progressively rise in the air and rotate upward around the elbows as the flexors increasingly contract and bend the arms over the chest, the hands clench into fists. At the end of the decorticate rigidity, the arms are flexed up in the air. After the release of the postural attitude, both arms slowly fall overhead by gravity, the palms of the hands facing upward; the arms reach their final position lying over the head on the floor at 2 min 33 s. Three isolated sudden muscular contractions (spasms) are observed at 3 min 15 s, 3 min 52 s, and 4 min 46 s. The body then remains motionless for the rest of the video.

Implications for toxicology and pathology

Human studies on the toxicity of propane are limited. Two studies of volunteers are available. In 1929, a study by Patty and Yant was mainly aimed at evaluating the odor detection of various alkanes, including propane.[21] Physiological responses and symptoms were only briefly described. No symptoms were reported for exposure of 10,000 ppm for 10 min, but vertigo was suffered for exposure of 100,000 ppm for 2 min. Neither loss of consciousness nor serious symptoms or sequelae was observed. In 1977, in a study by Stewart et al., volunteers were exposed to propane in three different conditions: 1,000 ppm for up to 10 min, 250 to 500 ppm for up to 8 min, and 1,000 ppm for 8 h per day for 9 days over 2 weeks.[22] Clinical parameters of heart, brain, lung, and adrenocortical functions were monitored, along with neurobehavioral parameters. No effects of the exposure to propane were found, and no symptoms were reported by the volunteers.

A few postmortem studies of lethal exposure to propane have been conducted.[23–25] In a case reported by Haq and Hameli,[23] it was found that the relative concentration of propane was higher in the brain, followed in order by the liver, lung, blood, and kidney. In the work of Graefe et al.,[24] the highest levels of propane in two fatal cases were 1,100 μg/ml in blood, 1,028 μg/g in lung, 820 μg/g in brain, 572 μg/g in liver, and 256 μg/g in kidney. Lower concentrations were reported by Pragst et al.[25]: 720 μg/ml in blood, 230 μg/ml in lung, and 120 μg/ml in brain.

In animal studies, cardiac sensitization has been observed in dogs following exposure to propane.[26–28] Cardiac sensitization is defined as the increased sensitity of the heart to epinephrine (endogenous or exogenous) after exposure to an organic chemical.[29] Cardiac sensitization is associated with cardiac arrhythmias and a risk of sudden death.

Since there are no studies to clearly establish the mechanism of death in propane-associated asphyxiation in humans, several mechanisms have been proposed. If indirect acute deaths by trauma or aspiration of vomit are excluded, four mechanisms of direct acute deaths have been proposed: anoxia, vagal inhibition, respiratory depression, and cardiac arrhythmia.[30,31] First, it is proposed that propane itself might not be toxic. Asphyxia could be related to direct displacement of oxygen either by propane or, in gas inhalation using a plastic bag, by rebreathing and the buildup of carbon dioxide.[32,33] Second, in inhalation with direct spraying of the gas inside the mouth, the release of high-pressure gas could produce freezing of the pharyngolaryngeal area, causing a reflex cardiac arrest by vagal inhibition.[30,32] Third, the hypothesis that seems to be favored by most authors is that propane could be toxic and cause respiratory depression with respiratory arrest or cardiac sensitization with arrhythmias and sudden cardiac arrest.[30–33]

The present case was the first reported fatal event with video recording; therefore, it provides tremendous new insight on propane-associated death. The comparison of the agonal sequence documented in the video to the agonal sequence observed in film recordings of other types of asphyxia is particularly interesting. There are two limitations to this comparison. First, the concentration of propane inhaled in this case is unknown. Second, it is probable that the agonal sequence in propane-related death will somehow vary depending on the concentration of propane in the inhaled air, but the extent of this concentration-related variation is unknown at this time. Despite these two limitations, the comparison of agonal sequences is nevertheless instructive.

In this present case of propane-associated asphyxiation, the agonal sequence witnessed led to a significantly faster death than in two documented cases of suffocation by plastic bag (see the section on the new data on smothering from the Working Group on Human Asphyxia). Loss of consciousness occurred in 32 s, followed by convulsions in 36 s, whereas in nonlethal recordings of suffocation by plastic bag (with moderately heavy and thick plastic bags only slightly bigger than the head), consciousness was not lost after 2 min 4 s in one case and 3 min in the other.

A comparison of the agonal sequence in hanging[15,16] reveals that the early responses in this propane-related death were strikingly similar, but delayed by 14 to 22 s: Loss of consciousness, convulsions, onset of deep rhythmic abdominal respiratory movements, and decorticate rigidity were all observed approximately 20 s later than in hanging deaths (Table 5.2). As for the late responses, the timing of both the end of deep rhythmic abdominal respiratory movements and the last muscle movement were in the usual distribution found in hanging (end of deep abdominal respiratory movements at 1 min 33 s in the propane case compared to an average of 1 min 51 s ± 30 s in hanging; and last muscle movement at 4 min 46 s in the propane case compared to an average of 4 min 12 s ± 2 min 29 s in hanging).

The striking similarity between propane-related death and hanging is in favor of a mechanism of death mainly based on an asphyxia process with oxygen replacement and depletion. Death by a toxic effect with cardiac sensitization seems less probable, at

Table 5.2 Comparison of Agonal Sequence in Propane-Related Asphyxiation and Hangings

	Propane-related asphyxiation	Average time in hanging (14 cases)[a]
Loss of consciousness	32 s	10 ± 3 s
Convulsions	36 s	14 ± 3 s
Decerebrate rigidity	Not observed	19 ± 5 s
Start of deep rhythmic abdominal respiratory movements	33 s	19 ± 5 s
Decorticate rigidity	58 s	38 ± 15 s
Loss of muscle tone	2 min 4 s	1 min 17 s ± 25 s
End of deep rhythmic abdominal respiratory movements	1 min 33 s	1 min 51 s ± 30 s
Last muscle movement	4 min 46 s	4 min 12 s ± 2 min 29 s

[a] From Sauvageau A, LaHarpe R, King D et al. *Am J Forensic Med Pathol* 2011;32(2):104–107.

least in this case. Further research is needed, and other filmed autoerotic accidents by gas mixtures should be analyzed.

Implications for crime scene interpretation

Another instructive point of this case report is the modification of the body position at the scene during the agonal sequence. It is well known by forensic experts that the position of the body at the scene is of tremendous importance in homicide investigation.[34,35] If the final position of the body at the crime scene seems unexpected or unusual when analyzed in relation to the cause of death or the dynamic of the altercation, postmortem moving of the body will be considered likely. This moving of the body could have been done for practical reasons, such as hiding the body or dumping the body elsewhere, or to stage the scene to make it appear to be something else, such as a suicide or an accident.[35] Rarely, the body could have been placed in a sexually degrading position, either to shock others or for the killer's own pleasure.[35]

If a victim was found with arms overhead in a strangulation case, it would generally be assumed that this body position was not the initial position at the time of the strangulation, and that therefore the body was moved afterward, either dragged by the arms or staged or posed in some way. The present case is the first to demonstrate that the arms can significantly change position during the agonal sequence in asphyxiation deaths, but a similar phenomenon had been previously observed in the legs.[36] In a filmed event, a man was hanging kneeling in a forward bent position. During the decorticate rigidity, his legs suddenly extended and remained extended thereafter.

To avoid wrongful interpretation of crime scenes, it is essential that crime scene specialists and criminal profilers are informed of this possible change of position of arms and legs during the agonal sequence in deaths by asphyxia.

Typical methods of autoerotic deaths: Checklist for the forensic expert

- Know that hanging constitutes the most widely used method of autoerotic practice (70% to 80% of autoerotic deaths).
- Know that plastic bags and chemical substances are the second most common method of autoerotic practice (10% to 30% of autoerotic deaths).

Definitions of terms: Checklist for the forensic expert

- Classify asphyxia by plastic bags and chemical substances as a subtype of suffocation.

Autoerotic deaths by smothering by plastic bags over the head: Checklist for the forensic expert

- In a scene of suffocation by plastic bag, take particular care to describe and document the type of plastic bag; the position of the bag in relation to the head, mouth, and nose; if the plastic bag is secured at the neck; if a ligature is present to enclose the bag; the type of ligature, its loops and knots; and the knots on the plastic bags.
- Do not remove the plastic bag from the head before proper photographic documentation if the victim is obviously dead.

- Be aware that without proper scene information, the diagnosis of smothering on a plastic bag over the head is likely to be missed.
- Know that the autopsy findings are nonspecific.

Autoerotic deaths by suffocation on chemical substances: Checklist for the forensic expert

- Know that the most commonly used chemical compounds in the context of autoerotic practice are hydrocarbons, anesthetic compounds, and other chemical inhalants.
- Pay particular attention to odors when entering a scene.
- At the scene, describe the presence of a gas tank, mask, plastic bag, or item of clothing on the face or head of the victim or beside the body.
- Know that plastic bags possibly containing chemicals can be submitted for toxicology (bags should be put in an airtight can or glass jar [no plastic container should be used] and refrigerated).
- Be aware that pressurized cans found at the scene should be seized for toxicological analysis.
- Be aware that some suffocation gases (e.g., helium) cannot be tested, and that scene investigation is extremely important to establish the cause of death.

References

1. Sauvageau A, Racette S. Autoerotic deaths in the literature from 1954 to 2004: a review. *J Forensic Sci* 2006;51(1):140–146.
2. Behrendt N, Modvig J. The lethal paraphiliac syndrome—accidental autoerotic death in Denmark 1933–1990. *Am J Forensic Med Pathol* 1995;16(3):232–237.
3. Blanchard R, Huscker SJ. Age, transvestism, bondage, and concurrent paraphilic activities in 117 fatal cases of autoerotic asphyxia. *Br J Psychiatry* 1991;159:371–377.
4. Diamond M, Innala SM, Ernulf KE. Asphyxiophilia and autoerotic death. *Hawaii Med J* 1990;49(1):11–12, 14–16, 24.
5. Sauvageau A. Autoerotic deaths: a 25-year retrospective epidemiological study. *Am J Forensic Med Pathol* 2012;33(2):143–146.
6. Sauvageau A, Boghossian E. Classification of asphyxia: the need for standardization. *J Forensic Sci* 2010;55(5):1259–1267.
7. Boghossian E, Tambuscio S, Sauvageau A. Non-chemical suffocation deaths in forensic setting: a 6-year retrospective study of environmental suffocation, smothering, choking and traumatic/positional asphyxia. *J Forensic Sci* 2010;55(3):646–651.
8. DiMaio VJ, DiMaio D. Asphyxia. In: Geberth VJ (series editor). *Forensic Pathology*, 2nd ed. Boca Raton, FL: CRC Press, 2001:229–277.
9. Spitz WU. Asphyxia. In: Spitz WU, Spitz DJ (eds), *Spitz and Fisher's Medicolegal Investigation of Death: Guidelines for the Application of Pathology to Crime Investigation*, 4th ed. Springfield, IL: Thomas, 2006:783–845.
10. Shkrum MJ, Ramsay DA. Asphyxia. In: Karch SB (series editor), *Forensic Pathology of Trauma: Common Problems for the Pathologist*. Totowa, NJ: Humana Press, 2007:65–179.
11. Saukko P, Knight B. Suffocation and "asphyxia." In: Ueberberg A (project editor). *Knight's Forensic Pathology*, 3rd ed. London: Arnold, 2004:352–367.
12. Jones LS, Wyatt JP, Busuttil A. Plastic bag asphyxia in southeast Scotland. *Am J Forensic Med Pathol* 2000; 21(4):401–405.
13. Rosen CL, Frost JD, Bricker T, Tarnow JD, Gillette PC, Dunlavy S. Two siblings with recurrent cardiorespiratory arrest: Munchausen syndrome by proxy or child abuse? *Pediatrics* 1983;71(5):715–720.

14. Sauvageau A, Ambrosi C, Kelly S. Autoerotic non-lethal filmed hangings: a case series and comments on the estimation of the time to irreversibility in hanging. *Am J Forensic Med Pathol* 2012;33(2):159–162.
15. Sauvageau A, LaHarpe R, Geberth VJ. Agonal sequences in eight filmed hangings: analysis of respiratory and movement responses to asphyxia by hanging. *J Forensic Sci* 2010; 55(5):1278–1281.
16. Sauvageau A, LaHarpe R, King D, Dowling G, Andrews S, Kelly S, Ambrosi C, Guay JP, Geberth VJ. The Working Group on Human Asphyxia. Agonal sequences in fourteen filmed hangings with comments on the role of the type of suspension, ischemic habituation and ethanol intoxication on the timing of agonal responses. *Am J Forensic Med Pathol* 2011;32(2):104–107.
17. Sauvageau A, Ambrosi C, Kelly S. Three non-lethal ligature strangulations filmed by an autoerotic practitioner: Comparison of early agonal responses in strangulation by ligature, hanging and manual strangulation. *Am J Forensic Med Pathol* 2012;33(4):339–340.
18. Evironmental Protection Agency. *Propane. Interim Acute Exposure Guideline Levels (AEGLs) for NAS/COT Subcommittee for AEGLS.* 2009. http://www.epa.gov/oppt/aegl/pubs/propane_interim_dec_2008.pdf (accessed October 20, 2010).
19. Isenschmid DS, Cassin BJ, Hepler BR, Kanluen S. Tetrachloroethylene intoxication in an autoerotic fatality. *J Forensic Sci* 1998;43(1):231–234.
20. Jones LS, Wyatt JP, Busuttil A. Plastic bag asphyxia in southeast Scotland. *Am J Forensic Med Pathol* 2000;21(4):401–405.
21. Patty FA, Yant WP. Odor intensity and symptoms produced by commercial propane, butane, pentane, hexane, and heptane vapor. *U.S. Bureau of Mines Report of Investigation* 1929;2979:1–10.
22. Stewart RD, Hermann AA, Baretta ED, Foster HV, et al. *Acute and Repetitive Human Exposure to Isobutene and Propane.* Report no. CTFA-MCOW-ENV-MBP-77-1. Springfield, VA: National Clearinghouse for Federal Scientific and Technical Information, 1977.
23. Haq MZ, Hameli AZ. A death involving asphyxiation from propane inhalation. *J Forensic Sci* 1980;25(1):25–28.
24. Graefe A, Müller RK, Vock R, Trauer H, Wehran HJ. Tödliche Intoxikationen durch Propan-Butan. *Arch Kriminol* 1999;203(1–2):27–31.
25. Pragst F, Prügel M, Vogel J, Herre S. Investigation of two fatal cases caused by inhalation of propane and chloroethane. *Schmiedeberg's Arch Pharmacol* 1991;344(Suppl 2):R127.
26. Krantz JC, Jr, Carr CJ, Vitcha JF. Anesthesia; a study of cyclic and noncyclic hydrocarbons on cardiac automaticity. *J Pharmacol Exp Ther* 1948;94(3):315–318.
27. Reinhardt CF, Azar A, Maxfield ME, Smith PE, Jr, Mullin LS. Cardiac arrhythmias and aerosol "sniffing." *Arch Environ Health* 1971;22(2):265–279.
28. Clark DG, Tinston DJ. Acute inhalation toxicity of some halogenated and non-halogenated hydrocarbons. *Hum Toxicol* 1982;1(3): 239–247.
29. Brock WJ, Rusch GM, Trochimowicz HJ. Cardiac sensitization: methodology and interpretation in risk assessment. *Regul Toxicol Pharmacol* 2003;38(1):78–90.
30. Shepherd RT. Mechanism of sudden death associated with volatile substance abuse. *Hum Toxicol* 1989;8(4):287–391.
31. Jackowski C, Römhild W, Aebi B, Bernhard W, Krause D, Dirnhofer R. Autoerotic accident by inhalation of propane-butane gas mixture. *Am J Forensic Med Pathol* 2005;26(4):355–359.
32. Saukko P, Knight B. Deaths from organic solvents. In: Ueberberg A (project editor), *Knight's Forensic Pathology*, 3rd ed. London: Arnold, 2004:595–599.
33. Fonseca CA, Auerbach DS, Suarez RV. The forensic investigation of propane gas asphyxiation. *Am J Forensic Med Pathol* 2002;23(2):167–169.
34. Geberth VJ. *Practical Homicide Investigation: Tactics, Procedures, and Forensic Techniques*, 4th edition. Boca Raton, FL: CRC Press, 2006.
35. Keppel RD, Weis JG. The rarity of "unusual" [corrected] dispositions of victim bodies: staging and posing. *J Forensic Sci* 2004;49(6):1308–1312.
36. Sauvageau A, Godin A, Desnoyers S, Kremer C. Six-year retrospective study of suicidal hangings: determination of the pattern of limb lesions induced by body responses to asphyxia by hanging. *J Forensic Sci* 2009;54(5):1089–1092.

chapter six

Atypical methods of autoerotic deaths

Introduction

The vast majority of autoerotic deaths are related to hangings (approximately 70% to 80%), followed by plastic bag and chemical substances (10% to 30%). However, it is important to keep in mind that other types of autoerotic deaths also exist: electrocution, overdressing/body wrapping, foreign body insertion, and atypical asphyxia methods.[1,2] These atypical autoerotic deaths, probably accounting for 5% to 10% of cases,[1,3] are often missed because police investigators, pathologists, or other forensic experts are not aware of their existence. To restrict autoerotic deaths as only asphyxia by hanging and plastic bags is unfortunately a common mistake.

Electrocution

Electricity is sometimes used by autoerotic practitioners for sexual stimulation. This is a dangerous practice that can lead to death by electrocution.

Deaths by electrocution can be divided into five types: low-voltage direct current, low-voltage alternating current, high-voltage direct current, high-voltage alternating current, and lightning.[4] In autoerotic deaths, electrocution usually involves low-voltage alternating current since most autoerotic practitioners simply use domestic current.

The electric system utilized for autoerotic stimulation is generally self-made. The electrical gadgetry often includes a voltage regulator or a prop that allows a deliberate variation of the current flow. Deaths are related either to a malfunction of the electrical device or to accidental contact with a more active part of the circuit. The mechanism of death is a lethal cardiac arrhythmia.

The electricity is used to stimulate the nipples, the scrotum, the penis, or the anorectal region. The thinness of the skin in the genital area and the mucosal surface may be a contributing factor in death by low-voltage electrocution.

Interestingly, rectal application of electricity is a known veterinary practice to obtain semen from bulls.[5] An electrode is connected to the rectal area and another to the sacral area, or a bipolar rectal electrode is used. The electric current produces an erection and an ejaculation in bulls. It was suggested that this may be the origin of electrical stimulation as an autoerotic practice.[5]

Examples from the literature

Sivaloganathan described the case of a 36-year-old television engineer, found dead in the flat he shared with his homosexual partner.[6] The body was found lying facedown on the floor of the combined kitchen and living room. A wire cradle had been applied to the scrotum, and another loop of wire had been inserted, with the end folded, into the anus. The wires were connected to the speakers of a television set, the back of which had been removed.

These wires, when switched on, could carry a current of approximately 0.6 A at 2.2 V. At autopsy, an electric burn was noticed on the right side of the face at the external corner of the right eye. The examination of the scene revealed that one of the wires had broken off. It seems that on cessation of all electrical stimulation activity, the man looked inside the back of the television to see what was wrong. In the process of this electric investigation, the right side of the face of the victim came in contact with the exposed metal cap of a valve (10 A of current at 2,500 V), and this current killed him. The shield usually covering the valve had been earlier removed by the victim in installing the electric stimulation apparatus.

Cairns and Rainer reported two cases of death from electrocution during autoerotic practice.[7] A 26-year-old qualified radio serviceman was found dead on the floor of his bedroom. Straps were surrounding his legs, and ropes were extending from his ankles to his wrists at the back of his knees. Underwear was stuffed in his mouth. The man was wearing a condom and had ejaculated into it. A potentiometer was installed on a dressing table, connected to two transformers supplying electricity through a three-pin plug. From the potentiometer, one wire extended beneath the deceased's clothing to his chest, where it was connected to two short leads soldered to 10-cent coins and taped to both nipples. The return wire was connected to another potentiometer that had been inserted into his rectum. Laboratory analyses revealed that the first transformer gave an output of 7.5 V, which was then connected to the second transformer for an output of 113.2 V. The potentiometer allowed varying this output from 0 to a maximum of 113.2 V. At autopsy, electrical burns were found on the nipples and rectum.

The other case described by Cairns and Rainer was a 58-year-old divorced man found dead in his flat at the top of an internal staircase.[7] The body was naked, with a wooden clamp around the chest creating fake breasts by compressing the soft tissue of the anterior chest wall. Items of female clothing were noticed at the scene. At autopsy, both nipples and the anus presented electrical burns. The scene investigation revealed that the decedent had used a ceiling light controlled by a dimmer switch as an electrical supply. The wires of the light were disconnected from the ceiling light and connected instead to the outlet socket of a cable extension lead. The cable extension lead was then connected to a three-pin plug while a three-core asbestos flex was connected to the plug by twisting the red and green wires around the phase pin and the black wire around the neutral pin. The other ends of the red and green wires were taped to 1-cent pieces on each nipple. The black wire was connected to a cylindrical metal electrode inserted in the anus. Depending on the position of the dimmer switch, the current varied from 0.35 to 230 V.

Cooke et al. published the case of a 32-year-old, found naked on his bed in the single-man quarters of a mining company.[8] It seems that the man had learned about electrical stimulation during a recent trip and failed to realize that the electric voltage on his trip was less than half that of his mining town (110 V compared to 240 V). At the scene, a metal neck chain was connected to the wires of an electric cord connected to a wall-mounted electric plug. The electric cord had been taken from an electric appliance; the appliance plug had been removed and the bare wires exposed. The metal chain, connected to the live wire, was wrapped around the penis of the deceased. The negative wire was in contact with the chest of the victim; the ground wire was tucked in the rubber shroud of the cord. At autopsy, electrical burns were found on the chest and around the penis. An assessment of the electric apparatus revealed that the amount of current flow could be changed by making contact with various parts of the metal chain, the distal part providing less stimulation than the proximal ones.

In another report by Klintschar et al., a 27-year-old man was found dead in his bedroom, lying on the floor, facedown on a blanket.[5] The body was nude except for a tennis sock placed over the penis. Electrical burns were found near the left nipple and on the right hand. The parents of the deceased tried to conceal the scene, but pornographic sado-masochistic material was found along with a bottle covered in feces. An electrical wire was also noticed, with separated strands connected to two self-made electrodes and with one of these electrodes connected to a tampon-shaped object. It was suggested that the latter electrode was initially inserted in the anus while the other was probably looped around the penis. The scene reconstruction and the autopsy findings suggested that after inserting one electrode in his anus, the deceased inadvertently touched the other with his right hand while trying to install it to his penis. A circuit from the penis to the anus would have spared the heart, but an electric circuit between the hand and the anus caused a heart fibrillation and death by electrocution.

An article by Schott et al. presented the case of an 18-year-old man found dead on his bed.[9] The man was wearing two bras and two pairs of men's briefs, attached at the crotch areas by plastic ties. A third pair of briefs was folded and inserted between the other two pairs, smoothing the genital area. The man was also wearing a short-sleeve T-shirt under-neath a tank-top shirt. The shirts were attached to the brassieres by plastic ties, causing the T-shirt to fold horizontally at the breast area. Pornographic material, with pictures of nude women, was recovered at the scene near the body. The bras were fashioned with metal washers and moist washcloths positioned within each cup. The exposed wires of an elec-tric cord were wrapped around the washers inside the bras. At autopsy, electrical burns were noticed on the mammary regions bilaterally.

Another typical case can be found in a study by Shields et al.[10] The body of a 39-year-old man was discovered in the back room of a synagogue. The man, a fugitive, was allowed to live there while the usual occupant was out of town. The deceased was clad in a female's negligee and stockings. The external genitalia were exposed. A pornographic book entitled *Tri County Swingers* was found near the body, and numerous enemas and douches were scattered throughout the room. A rheostat was connected to a 220-V electri-cal plug and to a wire attached to an inflatable catheter inserted into the victim's rectum. At autopsy, electrical burns of the left hand were documented, as well as intense erythema of the rectal mucosa.

Overdressing/body wrapping

Overdressing and body wrapping is an unusual autoerotic method that can potentially be dangerous and lethal. In these cases, the autoerotic practitioner has either piled up several layers of clothing or wrapped himself from almost head to toe in covering such as plastic bags or blankets. Death can be caused by different mechanisms, depending on the circum-stances. In some cases, the body wrapping covers the nose and mouth, causing death by smothering. In other cases, there is no impediment to breathing, and death is secondary to the hyperthermia associated with the multilayer overdressing or body wrapping.

Although it is difficult to understand the motivation to wrap oneself entirely in plastic or blankets, it seems that this practice might be linked to a desire to be enclosed or confined, and that this wish might be linked to a subconscious fantasy to return to the womb.[11]

Examples from the literature

In 1960, Johnstone et al. reported two cases of autoerotic asphyxia in relation to body wrapping and overdressing.[12] The first case was a 23-year-old schoolteacher, found dead wedged in a tall dustbin in a closet at his workplace. Women's shoes and theatrical grease paints and makeup were recovered at the scene, along with a homemade wooden box mask with holes for the neck, eyes, and mouth. The body was dressed with a plastic mackintosh over three cotton skirts, a thin rubberized raincoat, and a home-made plastic suit with holes for arms and neck. A sheet of plastic curtain was wrapped between the legs and around the abdomen. Seminal fluid was found on this plastic sheet. Fake breasts from towels were strapped over the chest. On the head, a woman's plastic rain cap was pulled over a rubber bathing cap. The face was covered by a thick layer of motor grease and hidden behind a net curtain and a polythene sheet with holes for mouth and eyes. The body was inserted head down in a tight bin. The second case was a 46-year-old engineer found dead in the closet of a public lavatory known to be frequented by homosexuals. The body was fully and properly dressed but wrapped from head to toe in a large, thin, transparent dry-cleaning plastic bag of about 6 x 4 ft (1.8 x 1.2 m).

Twenty-five years later, in 1985, another case was reported by Minyard[13]: A 34-year-old security guard was found at his workplace in a warehouse. The body was tightly wrapped in several layers of thin plastic similar to the thin plastic used by cleaners to cover clothing. Underneath the plastic, the body was nude except for a rubber hat. The head was also covered by the plastic, but the man used a snorkel device to breathe. The scene examination revealed that the man was masturbating when the snorkel fell from his mouth. The man tried to cut himself out of the wrapping by a pocketknife in his left hand, but he died of asphyxia before being able to cut his way out.

Eriksson et al. reported a case of body wrapping in blankets.[14] A 60-year-old man was found dead in his apartment, arms over head, rolled in 14 different blankets partially sewn together. Underneath the blankets, the body was clad in two pairs of hot pants, one pair of long johns, socks, and an undervest. His penis was thrust in a plastic bag containing paper with seminal fluid. It was noticed at the scene that the body was wet. The cause of death was attributed to asphyxia with a possible combination with hyperthermia. According to the scene reconstruction, the man piled up the blankets and fixed long strips of adhesive tape to the most external blankets. When he rolled himself up, the tape fixed the blankets together. The investigation revealed that the decedent purchased an astonishing number of blankets by mail order over the last few years (about 60 blankets were found in the apartment). The room where he was found was not furnished and was empty except for the blankets. Several floor markings from adhesive tape were documented, suggesting repetitive behavior. It seems that the man never allowed anyone in this room, alleging it was for workouts.

Madea described the case of a 56-year-old male found hanging head down in a sack.[15] The nude man, standing on two chairs, entered a sack head first. Tennis balls were tied to the free end of the sack, compressing his genitals. The sack was knotted to a board laid over a door and cupboard. The scene reconstruction revealed that one chair overturned. Because the center of gravity of the body was below the attached point, the body flipped head down. The man had scissors in his right hand, but after cutting a 15-cm opening in the sack, the fibers impacted between the blades and prevented further cutting action. Unable to get out of this precarious situation, the man died in the head-down position.

The case of a 46-year-old man who died of hyperthermia was reported by Byard et al.[16] The body was found in bushland, clad in a dress, women's undergarments, and seven pairs of stockings or pantyhose. The underwear had been cut to expose the genitals. The temperature where the body was found was higher than 39°C (70°F). Furthermore, the man was on benzotropine medical treatment, a drug known to have an atropine-like effect with anhydrosis and hyperthermia in hot weather.

A 34-year-old was found dead in his secured apartment.[11] The body, clad only in underwear, was completely enclosed from head to toe within a large plastic pocket (Figures 6.1a

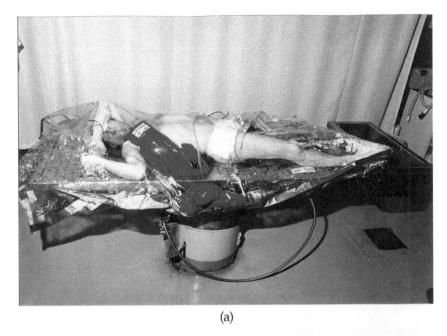

(a)

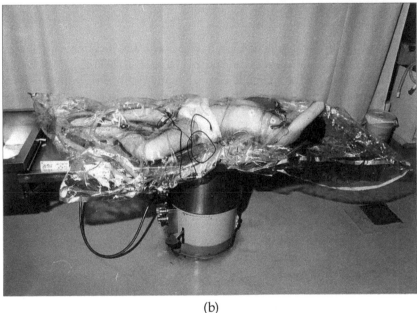

(b)

Figure 6.1 (a) and (b) Man found dead, completely enclosed from head to toe within a large plastic pocket. (From author Sauvageau files. Schellenberg, M., Racette, S., and Sauvageau, A., *J Forensic Sci* 207;52(4):954–956.)

and 6.1b). The plastic pocket had been made using a large plastic sheet folded in two and sealed on the remaining sides by duct tape, two from the outside and one from the inside. Red boxing gloves and a roll of duct tape were found along with the body. The plastic pocket was pierced by four tubes and a black wire, with three of the tubes obstructed by duct tape (Figure 6.2). Therefore, the only fresh air supply once inside the pocket was from

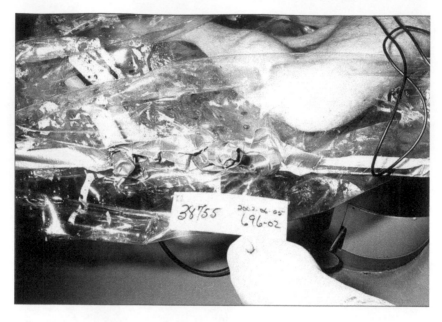

Figure 6.2 The plastic pocket was pierced by tubes, but only one tube was unobstructed by duct tape. (From author Sauvageau's files. Courtesy of editor, *Journal of Forensic Science*.)

the unobstructed tube approximately 1 cm in diameter. The internal portion of this tube was resting on the chest of the decedent, near his face. Insufficient gas exchange between the sealed plastic pocket and the outside caused asphyxia in the confined space. At some point, chemical substances might have been used as well since a knotted red plastic bag was found inside the plastic pocket, along with an uncapped aerosol can of leather and suede protector. As for the black wire piercing the bag, it was plugged into a nearby computer and connected to headphones inside the pocket. Sadomasochistic content was on the computer, and numerous photographs of nude men were scattered next to the computer and throughout the apartment. The autopsy was unremarkable apart from pulmonary edema. Toxicological analyses revealed a blood alcohol level of 119 mg/100 ml and traces in the blood of the hydrocarbons naphtha and Varsol™.

Although it is difficult to understand the motivation of someone to wrap entirely in plastic or blankets, it seems that this practice might be linked to a desire to be enclosed or confined, and that this wish might be linked to a subconscious fantasy to return to the womb.[11] This case illustrates particularly well the subconscious fantasy to return to the womb that is thought to motivate some autoerotic practitioners to wrap themselves completely in enclosed, confined environments. The plastic pocket, with its tubes and wire, reproduces to some extent the womb environment with the placenta and the umbilical cord.

Case history: Body wrapped in plastic

The victim had been diagnosed with mild schizophrenia. He had failed to show up for work, and when friends went to his residence to check on him, they found him dead under bizarre circumstances and notified the police. The man was completely wrapped in Reynolds Wrap® plastic with duct tape over his entire head (Figures 6.3 through 6.6). Detectives found several other plastic suits of Reynolds Wrap and duct tape that the

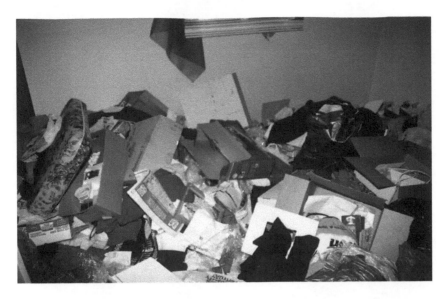

Figure 6.3 Cluttered apartment. This photo depicts the cluttered condition of the deceased's apartment, where the authorities recovered numerous plastic and duct tape remnants of outfits the deceased had worn. (Courtesy of Detective Mark Burbridge, Spokane, Washington, Police Department; submitted from author Geberth's files.)

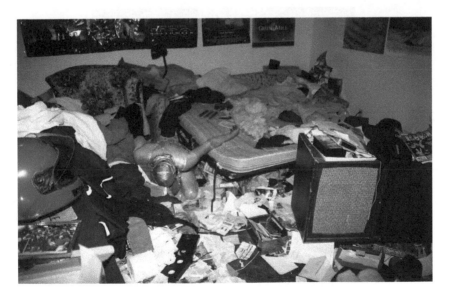

Figure 6.4 Victim in crime scene. This overview of the crime scene depicts the victim's body as it was found by arriving police officers. (Courtesy of Detective Mark Burbridge, Spokane, Washington, Police Department; submitted from author Geberth's files.)

victim had made on previous occasions and that he had cut off himself. It was hypothesized that the victim, who had wrapped himself in plastic, had his duct tape mask on and inadvertently knocked his scissors to the floor and could not find them prior to becoming unconscious. At the time of the case, detectives had developed the photos from a camera found in the scene. These pictures showed the victim taking photos of himself as he took steps to wrap himself. Several of the existing photos depicted

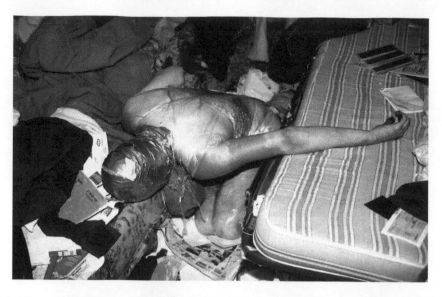

Figure 6.5 Close-up of victim's body. This close-up photo shows how the victim's body was completely wrapped in plastic with duct tape covering his head. (Courtesy of Detective Mark Burbridge, Spokane, Washington, Police Department; submitted from author Geberth's files.)

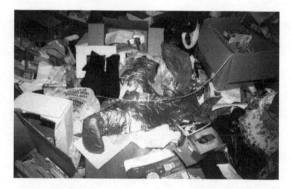

Figure 6.6 Plastic and duct tape suit. This photo depicts a partial outfit of plastic and duct tape that the victim had cut from his body from an earlier event. (Courtesy of Detective Mark Burbridge, Spokane, Washington, Police Department; submitted from author Geberth's files.)

wrapping with Ace™ bandages. Detectives speculated that the victim started with the Ace bandages and progressed to the Reynolds Wrap and duck tape.

Case history: Body completely wrapped in duct tape

This case, which occurred in an affluent suburb of Toledo, Ohio, was initially reported as a homicide by the small police department, which requested assistance from the Toledo Crime Scene Unit. Initially, the officers thought that the victim was a female due to the dark wig and nylon stockings. The actual crime scene was inside a private tennis club. The deceased was subsequently identified as the 64-year-old, white male tennis club manager. The body was found in the kitchen area on the first floor, near

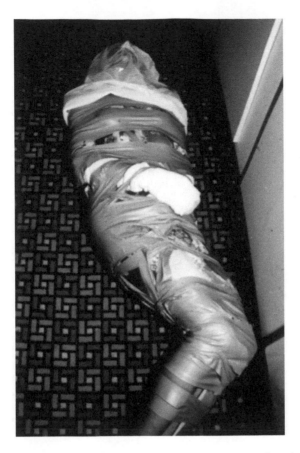

Figure 6.7 Victim at scene. This photo depicts how the victim appeared to the responding officers. He was completely wrapped in duct tape, with a plastic bag over his head, wearing nylon stockings and high-heel shoes. (Courtesy of Detective Terry Cousino, Toledo, Ohio, Police Department. Reprinted with permission from V. J. Geberth, *Sex-Related Homicide and Death Investigation: Practical and Clinical Perspectives,* 2nd edition, CRC Press, Boca Raton, FL, 2010, p. 130.)

the stairs to the small second-floor apartment where the club manager lived during the months warm enough for the club to be busy. The deceased actually had a wife at home in Michigan. Investigators immediately suspected the possibility that this case was an autoerotic death due to the cross-dressing and lack of any evidence of a break-in or physical assault. However, due to the extent to which the body was wrapped, the investigators initially believed that the victim, who was a willing participant, must have had some help (Figures 6.7 and 6.8). The crime scene investigators actually made a tent around the body and processed it with superglue fuming to attempt to find latent fingerprints of this possible "helper." The prints were all the victim's. When investigators went upstairs to the manager's apartment, they found ample evidence that the victim had in fact engaged in this autoerotic activity alone and further evidence that he apparently had done this many times previuosly. The victim's ritual included first dressing in women's clothing (including makeup). He put a Tylenol® bottle over his penis to catch the semen. He then wrapped ribbons and duct tape around his legs. Next, he wrapped his head, leaving only an opening to breathe through his nose. He also added a plastic garbage bag over his head. He then covered his hands with socks and duct tape. He then hopped to a doorway at the west end of his living room where he had rolls of

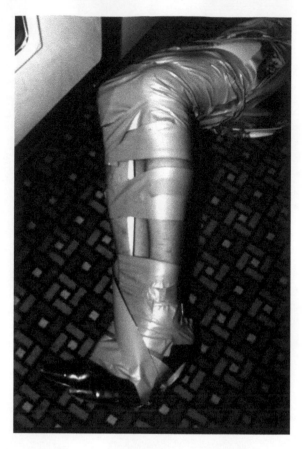

Figure 6.8 Extensive duct taping. This photo depicts the extensive amount of duct tape that the victim was able to wrap around himself at the scene. Note the high-heel shoes. (Courtesy of Detective Terry Cousino, Toledo, Ohio, Police Department; submitted from author Geberth's files.)

duct tape on toilet paper roll holders that were nailed to the door molding (Figure 6.9). There were numerous nail holes in the molding from prior events (Figure 6.10). Once he got the loose ends of the duct tape stuck to his body, he spun around until he was completely wrapped in duct tape. When he was ready to escape, he hopped to another doorway at the east end of his living room and used the ball ends of the empty hinge plates (the door was missing) to break the tape until he was loose enough to escape (there was a fairly large amount of duct tape adhesive residue around the ball ends of the hinge plates). Investigators learned from the suburban patrol officers that approximately 1 year earlier they had found the victim outside the tennis club tied up in ropes and seeking help. At the time, the victim explained to the officers that this was a practical joke that his friends had played on him.

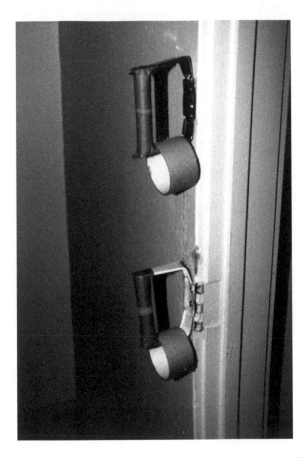

Figure 6.9 Duct tape rolls. The victim hopped to a doorway, where he had rolls of duct tape on toilet paper holders, which were nailed into door molding. (Courtesy of Detective Terry Cousino, Toledo, Ohio, Police Department. Reprinted with permission from V. J. Geberth, *Sex-Related Homicide and Death Investigation: Practical and Clinical Perspectives,* 2nd edition, CRC Press, Boca Raton, FL, 2010, p. 131.)

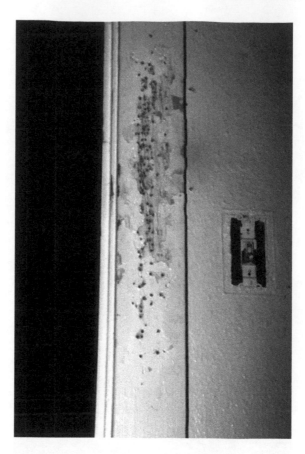

Figure 6.10 Nail holes: dozens of additional nail holes in the molding indicated habitual practice of body wrapping. (Courtesy of Detective Terry Cousino, Toledo, Ohio, Police Department. Reprinted with permission from V. J. Geberth, *Sex-Related Homicide and Death Investigation: Practical and Clinical Perspectives*, 2nd edition, CRC Press, Boca Raton, FL, 2010, p. 132.)

Case history: Body in canvas bag—chest compression

The victim, who was a psychologist at a state prison, had taken a canvas laundry bag from the prison to construct an unusual device (Figures 6.11a to 6.11d). Reportedly, he and his wife would play sex games together, including various BDSM (bondage, discipline, dominance/submission, sadomasochism) and S&M (sadomasochism) scenarios. He was supposed to wait for her to come home before engaging in any sexual activities involving bondage and deprivation of oxygen.

However, on this particular day the victim had decided to engage in some autoerotic activity. The victim used the large commercial laundry bag from his place of employment as a cocoon to envelop his body. He first wrapped himself in a large plastic bag before getting into the laundry bag. The victim planned to use the blower of a vacuum cleaner to inflate the plastic bag inside the canvas laundry bag. The victim, who was wearing his wife's teddy and nothing else, had apparently pulled the plastic bag and the laundry

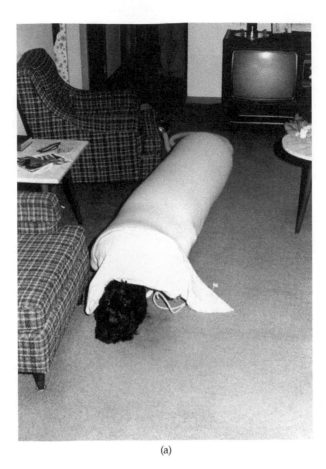
(a)

Figure 6.11 (a)–(d) The victim had used the blower end of a vacuum cleaner to inflate a plastic bag, which was inside a canvas laundry bag secured with a rope around his neck. (From author Geberth's files.)

bag up to his neck and was able to secure the bag by pulling the laundry bag ropes taut, which would trap the air inside the plastic bag. His arms were inside this contraption.

To turn the vacuum on, he had to roll over to the vacuum cleaner and turn it on with his nose. The blower of the vacuum cleaner then filled the plastic bag with air, which in turn caused the canvas bag to tighten around the subject's body. The laundry bag became as hard as a basketball, producing chest compression. During the crime scene investigation, the detectives turned off the vacuum cleaner, and the laundry bag and plastic bag inside immediately deflated. When the canvas bag was opened, they saw that the man was wearing his wife's lingerie.

The major problem with his contraption was that there was no way for the victim to turn off the vacuum once the canvas bag had become inflated. As the vacuum continued to pump air into the plastic bag, the man was not able to breathe due to chest and abdominal compression.

(b)

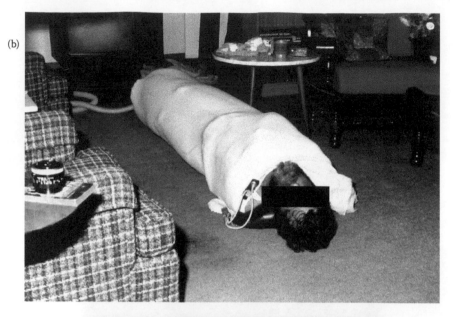

(c)

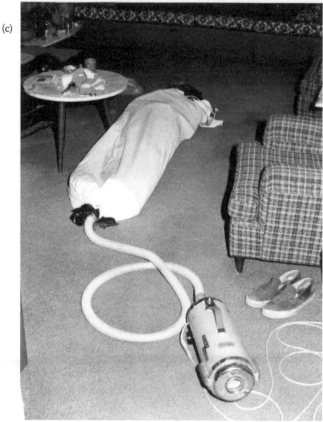

Figure 6.11 (continued) (a)–(d) The victim had used the blower end of a vacuum cleaner to inflate a plastic bag, which was inside a canvas laundry bag secured with a rope around his neck. (From author Geberth's files.)

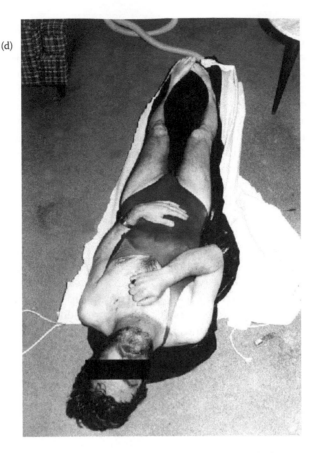

Figure 6.11 (continued) (a)–(d) The victim had used the blower end of a vacuum cleaner to inflate a plastic bag, which was inside a canvas laundry bag secured with a rope around his neck. (From author Geberth's files.)

Foreign body insertion

Foreign body insertion is often used in autoerotic practice as a means to enhance sexual pleasure. This sexual practice is usually innocuous. Extremely rarely, these autoerotic manipulations may cause an immediate or a delayed death. Immediate deaths by foreign body insertion can be related to acute hemorrhage, obstruction of the airways, or air embolism. Delayed deaths are usually associated with an infectious process secondary to the presence of a trapped foreign body or to a perforation of a hollow viscus. Delayed autoerotic deaths are challenging since the death scene is almost meaningless, and the correct assessment of the manner of death relies mainly on a thorough investigation. A common mistake would be to classify these cases as natural, overlooking their autoerotic accidental nature.

Examples from the literature

A 23-year-old man was found dead in his home.[17] Before his death, he had been complaining of weakness and fever, with chills and rigors. He was also complaining of having developed bedwetting in the 18 months prior to his death. He had consulted a doctor and had been treated with an antidepressant for this bedwetting. At autopsy, it was noticed that the body showed signs of dehydration. The kidneys showed bilateral pyelonephritis, and there was acute cystitis with a large stone filling the bladder (approximately 7.5 x 7.5 x 5 cm). On closer examination, a coiled plastic tube was found inside the stone. The tube, 3 mm in diameter, was estimated radiologically to measure approximately 20 to 30 cm long. Biochemical analyses confirmed that the decedent had developed renal insufficiency. The cause of death was superimposed bronchopneumonia on an acute pyelonephritis, due to a stone in the bladder, due to a foreign body. It was concluded after extensive inquiries that the tube had not been inserted for diagnostic or therapeutic procedures. It seems that the decedent introduced the tube for an autoerotic purpose some considerable time prior to death. The tube probably slipped from his hands and found its way into the bladder. Embarrassed, he did not seek medical attention.

A 40-year-old woman was discovered dead, lying naked on her bed.[18] A carrot was inserted into her vagina. The room was undisturbed, and there was no pornographic element at the scene. The external examination of the body was unremarkable apart from the inserted carrot. At autopsy, the heart was dissected under water after clamping of the vessels, revealing the presence of an air embolism in the heart cavities. Air was also found in the inferior vena cava; the lungs were heavy and congested. The carrot was 17 cm in length with a diameter varying from 2.5 to 4 cm from the tip to the base, respectively. The vagina and uterus were unremarkable apart from the presence of an intrauterine device (IUD); the site of the defect was not found. The cause of death was certified as air embolism secondary to vaginal insertion of a foreign body for an autoerotic purpose.

A 29-year-old man showed up at his neighbor's house early one afternoon, frantically knocking at the front door.[8] The man was holding his abdomen and was trying unsuccessfully to talk. He was then witnessed to collapse on the ground and died despite resuscitative efforts. At autopsy, a zucchini was found impacted in the larynx and oropharynx, totally obstructing the airways. The body was fully dressed, but the waist button of the pants was unfastened. A rubber band was noted around the base of the penis, and semen was noticed in the groin area.

A 40-year-old man was found dead.[16] He reportedly had been feeling unwell for the previous several days. It was found at autopsy that an unsharpened lead pencil had been introduced through the urinary tract and had perforated the bladder, causing fatal peritonitis. The pencil was found lying free in the abdominal cavity.

A 56-year-old man was found dead, lying naked in his bed.[16] At the scene, a large pool of blood was found on the floor beside the bed, with blood droplets in the hallway leading to the toilet and blood in the toilet bowl. A blood-stained shoe horn was found. At autopsy, a 3 cm traumatic tear was observed in the lower rectum and posterior anal canal, extending into the sphincter. The cause of death was attributed to hemorrhage due to an anal laceration from a shoehorn.

Case history: Body impaled—homemade device

A victim had constructed a long ceramic cone in the base of his "play toilet," which extended above the rim of the toilet seat (Figures 6.12a and 6.12b). Over the toilet, the subject had constructed a pulley system. He had affixed a wooden seat with a hole in the bottom that fit over the ceramic cone, which was lubricated with Vaseline®. He pulled himself up and down with the ropes on the pulleys. As the subject would lower himself over the toilet seat, the ceramic cone would go into his anal cavity. The subject apparently did not keep up with maintenance on his system, and one day one of the ropes, which was worn, broke. The subject was impaled on this device when discovered.

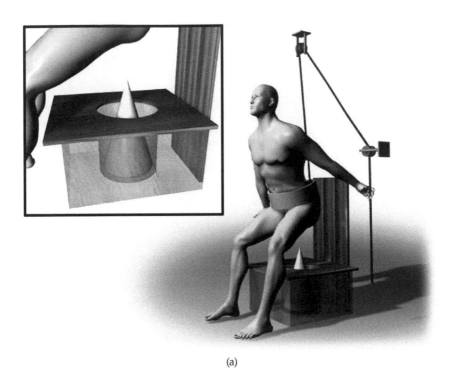

(a)

Figure 6.12 (a) and (b) Play toilet. Subject created this contraption for sexual gratification. The concept was to stimulate himself anally by riding up and down on the ceramic cone. He used a series of ropes and pulleys. The ropes became frayed and apparently snapped during one of his activities. (Courtesy of Medical Legal Art. Illustration copyright 2009 Medical Legal Art, http://www.doereport.com. Reprinted with permission from V. J. Geberth, *Sex-Related Homicide and Death Investigation: Practical and Clinical Perspectives*, 2nd edition, CRC Press, Boca Raton, FL, 2010, p. 128.)

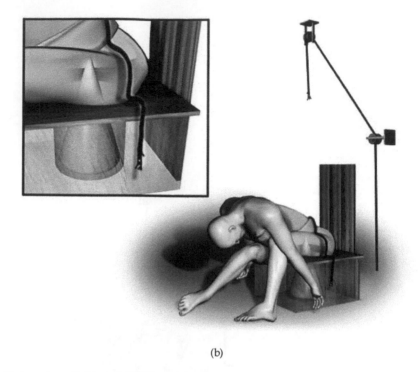

(b)

Figure 6.12 (continued) (a) and (b) Play toilet. Subject created this contraption for sexual gratification. The concept was to stimulate himself anally by riding up and down on the ceramic cone. He used a series of ropes and pulleys. The ropes became frayed and apparently snapped during one of his activities. (Courtesy of Medical Legal Art. Illustration copyright 2009 Medical Legal Art, http://www.doereport.com. Reprinted with permission from V. J. Geberth, *Sex-Related Homicide and Death Investigation: Practical and Clinical Perspectives,* 2nd edition, CRC Press, Boca Raton, FL, 2010, p. 128.)

Atypical asphyxia methods

Autoerotic asphyxias by hanging, plastic bag, and chemical substances are common and therefore considered typical asphyxia methods. All other types of asphyxia are classified as atypical asphyxia methods. Reported uncommon autoerotic asphyxia methods include ligature strangulation, chest compression, inverted or abdominal suspension, immersion and drowning, and smothering.

Definition of terms: The classification of asphyxia

The topic of asphyxia is a rather complex one, and a good understanding of the meaning of the various terms is important to avoid confusion. Unfortunately, the classification of asphyxia and the definition of subtypes are far from uniform, varying widely from one textbook to another and from one article to the next. Closely comparable cases are labeled differently by equally competent forensic pathologists. In an effort to standardize the classification of asphyxia, a unified model of classification was proposed in 2010.[19]

In this new standardized classification of asphyxia in the forensic context, four main categories of asphyxia are recognized: suffocation, strangulation, positional and traumatic asphyxia, and drowning (Figure 6.13). Suffocation includes three separates forms: smothering, choking, and confined spaces/entrapment/vitiated atmosphere. Strangulation also subdivides into three forms: ligature strangulation, hanging, and manual strangulation.

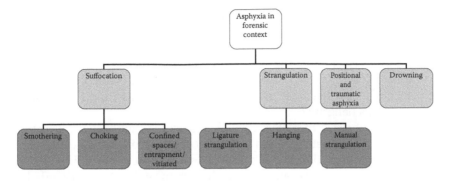

Figure 6.13 Classification of asphyxia in the forensic context.

Table 6.1 Definitions of Terms in the Proposed Unified Classification

Term	Definition
Suffocation	A broad term encompassing different types of asphyxia, such as vitiated atmosphere and smothering, associated with deprivation of oxygen
Smothering	Asphyxia by obstruction of the air passages above the epiglottis, including the nose, mouth, and pharynx
Choking	Asphyxia by obstruction of the air passages below the epiglottis
Confined spaces/ entrapment/ vitiated atmosphere	Asphyxia in an inadequate atmosphere by reduction of oxygen, displacement of oxygen by other gases, or by gases causing chemical interference with the oxygen uptake and utilization
Strangulation	Asphyxia by closure of the blood vessels or air passages of the neck as a result of external pressure on the neck
Ligature strangulation	A form of strangulation in which the pressure on the neck is applied by a constricting band tightened by a force other than body weight
Hanging	A form of strangulation in which the pressure on the neck is applied by a constricting band tightened by the gravitational weight of the body or part of the body
Manual strangulation	A form of strangulation caused by an external pressure on the structures of the neck by hands, forearms, or other limbs
Positional or postural asphyxia	A type of asphyxia in which the position of an individual compromises the ability to breathe
Traumatic asphyxia	A type of asphyxia caused by external chest compression by a heavy object
Drowning	Asphyxia by immersion in a liquid

The definitions of each entity are presented in Table 6.1. The majority of these subtypes of asphyxia have been described in the context of autoerotic asphyxia: hanging, ligature strangulation, smothering, choking, confined spaces and vitiated atmosphere, positional asphyxia, and drowning.

Ligature strangulation

In 2006, a review article concerning 50 years of literature on autoerotic deaths demonstrated that the most common methods of autoerotic activity leading to death were hanging, ligature, plastic bags, and chemical substances.[1] The recent standardization of the classification of asphyxia, however, had an impact on these conclusions, and ligature strangulation is no longer considered a common method of autoerotic activity.[2]

In the standardized classification of asphyxia, ligature strangulation is defined as a form of strangulation in which the pressure on the neck is applied by a constricting band tightened by a force other than the body weight.[19] If the pressure on the neck is applied by a constricting band tightened by the gravitational weight of the body or part of the body, the strangulation is classified as hanging.[19] With a strict application of these definitions, the vast majority of cases that were previously classified as ligature strangulation should now be reclassified as hanging.[2]

The first group of cases to reclassify includes victims who kneeled forward with a constricting band attached behind them to a bedpost or a doorknob. Because of the relative horizontality of the constricting band, these cases were previously classified as ligature strangulation. With a strict application of the definition of the standardized classification of asphyxia, these cases should now be reclassified as hangings since, despite the relative horizontality of the ligature, it was still the body weight that had tightened the constricting band around the neck.

The second group of cases to reclassify includes the victims that lay on their abdomen and tied their ankles or feet to their neck. These cases were previously classified as ligature strangulation. However, the asphyxia was caused by a constriction of the ligature around the neck by the weight of the legs; therefore, this is also a type of hanging. The fact that at some point there was a voluntarily movement to create the asphyxia is irrelevant: The victim stepping from a stool to hang has also done a voluntarily movement, and no one will contest that this is nevertheless a hanging.

After a critic review of all the previous cases classified as autoerotic ligature strangulation in the 50-year review study, only two cases were maintained as autoerotic ligature strangulation activity leading to death.[1,2] The first, described by Danto, was the case of a 21-year-old female found completely nude on the bathroom floor, kneeling at the bathtub, head underwater.[20] Doors were locked, and there were no signs of forced entry. Vomitus was noted in the water in the tub. A piece of sash cord was wrapped several times around her neck. A similar cord was wrapped around her wrists, without tying them. An iron bolt found under the victim's buttocks was thought to have been used for masturbation (Figure 6.14). An abrasion was observed on her forehead. After a long investigation, it was concluded that the victim was engaged in masturbation with autoerotic asphyxia by ligature when she lost consciousness and collapsed momentarily, striking her head against the side of the bathtub. The autoerotic method used in this case to enhance the sexual pleasure was ligature, since it was by actively holding a ligature on both sides of her neck that the victim created the asphyxia (the weight of the body or the weight of her arms was not the element here, but the active pulling of the extremities of the cord). After losing consciousness from the ligature strangulation, her face went into the water.

The other case was a 45-year-old woman found nude on the floor beside her bed.[21] An electric cord was looped around her neck and the bedpost. The extremities of the electric cord were wrapped several times to her right wrist. A nightgown wrapped around her neck ensured protective padding. She was controlling the tension on the ligature by actively pulling with her arms. The method of autoerotic asphyxia used here was therefore ligature strangulation. However, it seems that after her inadvertent loss of consciousness, the ligature became entangled tightly to the bedpost, and she died.

Interestingly, the only two cases of death following true ligature strangulation as a method of autoerotic practice were described in females. It is well known that females have a tendency to use less violent methods than males when committing suicides; by analogy, it can be hypothesized that females also prefer less violent methods in the inducing of autoerotic asphyxia. Compared to hanging, ligature strangulation appears less

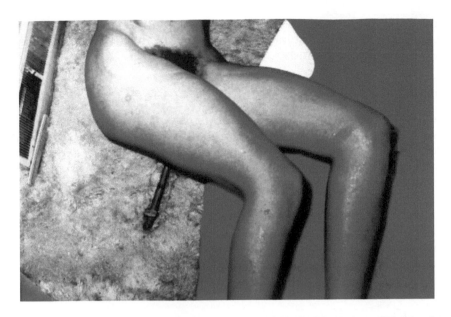

Figure 6.14 Female victim: atypical autoerotic. A metal bolt had been inserted into the victim's vagina from the rear. There was a rope secured around the victim's neck, and she was bent over the water-filled tub. At first, the case appeared to be a sex-related homicide. However, on closer examination it was revealed that the rope was loosely placed around the neck, and the deceased could control the pressure by pulling the end, which was in the front of her body. She apparently lost consciousness, and her face went into the water. (Courtesy of Supervisory Special Agent Robert R. Hazelwood, Behavioral Science Unit, FBI Academy, Quantico, Virginia, retired. Reprinted with permission from V. J. Geberth, *Practical Homicide Investigation: Tactics, Procedures and Forensic Techniques*, 4th edition, Boca Raton, FL, 2006, p. 375.)

threatening and is in fact less dangerous since the ending of voluntary movements following the loss of consciousness will interrupt the active pulling of the ligature around the neck.

Despite the absence of reported cases of autoerotic death following ligature strangulation in men, the nonlethal practice of ligature strangulation has been encountered. The Working Group on Human Asphyxia has reported the case of a 35-year-old man who filmed several of his autoerotic asphyxia sessions, including both hanging and ligature strangulation.[22] These films were found at the scene after his accidental death by hanging. In three filmed nonlethal ligature strangulations, the man is sitting on a chair. A pair of pajama pants is rolled once around his neck, with the extremities of the pants falling on each side of his chest. The man is pulling the extremities of the pants with both hands to apply compression on his neck. The man is seen to lose consciousness 11 s after the onset of strangulation and then to present convulsions. After losing consciousness, he ceases to pull on the ligature, and the pants slowly loosen around the neck. A few seconds later (16 to 18 s after the onset of strangulation), he regains consciousness and gets up from the chair.

Considering that the early agonal responses observed in these filmed ligature strangulations are highly similar to the ones detailed in hangings by the Working Group on Human Asphyxia,[23–25] it is thought that the later responses are similar as well. Therefore, the following agonal sequence is expected, with time 0 representing the onset of ligature strangulation: rapid loss of consciousness in 10 ± 3 s, mild generalized convulsions in 14 ± 3 s, decerebrate rigidity in 19 ± 5 s, beginning of deep rhythmic abdominal respiratory movements in 19 ± 5 s, decorticate rigidity in 38 ± 15 s, loss of muscle tone in 1 min 17 s ± 25 s, end of deep abdominal respiratory movements in 1 min 51 s ± 30 s, and last muscle movement in 4 min 12 s ± 2 min 29 s.

Chest compression

The autoerotic asphyxia method leading to death was attributed to chest compression in five cases. One of these cases was reported in a 14-year study among 117 compiled cases of autoerotic deaths.[26] The four other cases were mentioned as part of a review study of 70 cases.[27] In both articles, unfortunately, no detail was given regarding the specific method of chest compression.

Considering the new standardized classification of asphyxia, these cases are probably traumatic asphyxia by external chest compression by a heavy object. In some other instances, it is also possible that elaborate bondage maintained the victim in a position compromising the breathing movements (positional asphyxia). This is speculation, though, since there is no detailed case in the literature. Forensic experts are strongly encouraged, if coming across such cases, to report them as case reports.

Inverted or abdominal suspension

Autoerotic practitioners sometimes suspend themselves upside down (inverted position) or use a ligature to dangle in the air from their midsection (abdominal suspension). Although this practice is not as dangerous as hanging or electrocution, it encompasses risk of death by head down or death by positional asphyxia.

Deaths by head down are rare accidental events in which the victim is found in an inverted body posture with marked congestion of the face and dependent body parts and no definite pathoanatomical cause of death.[28] It is an exclusion diagnosis that can only be put forward after elimination of other possible causes of death, following a scene investigation, medical record review, complete autopsy, and toxicological analyses. It is important to remember that it is not merely because a victim is found head down that the final cause of death will be death by head down. Furthermore, this cause of death should not be confused with the more common positional asphyxia: In positional asphyxia, the position of the body interferes with the ability of the individual to breathe by restriction of the respiratory movements at the thoracic or abdominal level. In death by head down, there is no restriction of the ability to breathe, and there is no restriction of the respiratory movements of the thorax and abdomen. The physiopathology of death by head down is complex, but it seems that death is not related to asphyxia but to heart failure secondary to the increased burden of work for the heart in this unnatural position.[28]

O'Halloran and Dietz in 1993 published the first case of death in an autoerotic head-down position.[29] A 62-year-old man, nude except for 8-inch red high heels and knee-high nylon stockings, had his legs spread with the ankles secured on a pipe with duct tape. The pipe was suspended from a yoke fastened to the front-loader bucket of a tractor. Ropes were attached to the control lever of the tractor, allowing the victim to raise and tilt the bucket from a distance. It seems that the man used this system to suspend himself by the ankles in an inverted position. A 5-ft piece of 2 x 4 inch lumber was placed under the tractor scoop as a safety measure, preventing it from drifting down. Unfortunately, the lumber eventually snapped, and the scoop dropped, pinning the man down by pressing on his back. In this case, the autoerotic method used in the sexual fantasy was the head-down position, but the cause of death was traumatic asphyxia.

A 57-year study of autoerotic deaths in Denmark compiled 2 inverted suspension cases from 46 autoerotic deaths.[30] No details were available on these unusual cases.

A case of abdominal suspension, with death by positional asphyxia, was reported by Thibault et al.[31] A 27-year-old man was found dead in a storage room at work. The nude man was suspended from his midsection by an abdominal ligature. The abdominal ligature was tied by a rope to a hand-operated winch suspended by another rope to a steam pipe. Several marks on the pipe suggested previous similar activities. A shed behind his home, where his wife said he was spending a considerable amount of time, was found to be equipped with a grappling hook suspended by a steel cable to a crossbeam. Several notches were noted on the wooden crossbeam, and numerous semen stains were found in that shed.

Immersion and drowning

Immersion in water is a rare sexual pleasure enhancement activity. The first case of aqua eroticum was reported by Sivaloganathan.[32] A 36-year-old man was found dead at the bottom of a river. His right ankle was fastened by a clothesline to a large stone. The man was dressed in female clothes, with a bra stuffed to create breasts, and hair clips were attached to his nipples. The man was wearing makeup. A pair of scissors was on his right index finger by the small loop. Several other large stones with cut clothesline were found at the bottom of the river by police divers. This man was using immersion as an autoerotic method and died by drowning.

Case history: Immersion and drowning

Another aqua eroticum case was later reported.[33] The body of a 25-year-old man was found floating on a lake in summertime. The man was clad in a hockey helmet with a safety grid, a two-piece snowmobile suit, and beige ski boots (Figure 6.15). A complex bondage system made of horseback riding straps was circling the waist, tying together the

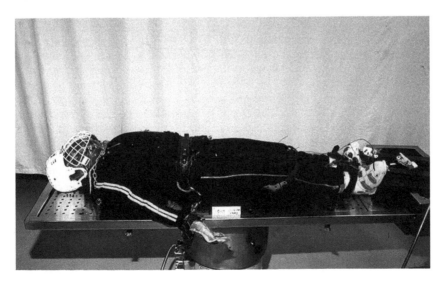

Figure 6.15 The decedent was found clad in a hockey helmet and a two-piece snowmobile suit and beige ski boots, with a complex bondage system. (From Sauvageau, A. and Racette, S. Courtesy of the editor, *J Forensic Sci* 2006;51(1):137–139.)

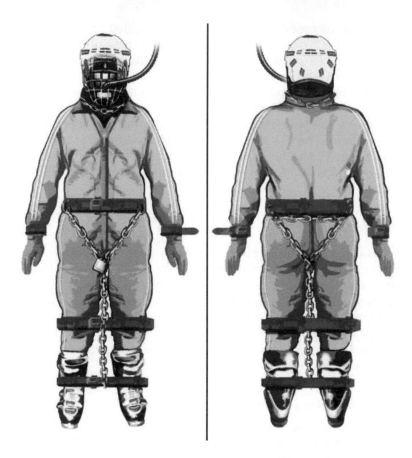

Figure 6.16 Complex bondage system made of horseback riding straps, chains, and padlock. (Courtesy of editor, *Journal of Forensic Science* and courtesy of Medical Legal Art. Illustration copyright 2009 Medical Legal Art, http://www.doereport.com.)

knees and fastening the ankles (Figure 6.16). Chains were tying these straps together, and the bondage system was secured at the pubic region by a padlock. Separate straps were found at each wrist, unattached to the rest of the chains and straps. Under the bondage system and the winter garments, the body was wrapped from head to toe in a transparent homemade plastic jumpsuit, with the opening at the front closed by duct tape (Figure 6.17). Over the face, a black plastic tube was sealed by silicone to the suit, allowing an air supply. Under the leakproof plastic suit, the body was naked, and a small piece of plastic was tied to the penis by an elastic. A scene reconstruction revealed that the victim was completely immersed in the water, with the ski boots on his feet connected by ski bindings to a wooden board attached to a floating pneumatic boat (Figure 6.18). The breathing tube sealed to the plastic jumpsuit was connected by a longer 4.5-m plastic tube to an open plastic container floating at the surface. This elaborate home-diving apparatus presented a major flaw: The victim was inhaling and exhaling through a tube too long to allow sufficient air exchange, with inhalation being mainly reinhalation of the carbon dioxide–laden exhaled air.

Apart from these two well-described aqua eroticum cases, another autoerotic drowning was briefly mentioned in a German study of 16 autoerotic deaths in the Hannover area.[34] Unfortunately, there were no details concerning this third autoerotic drowning.

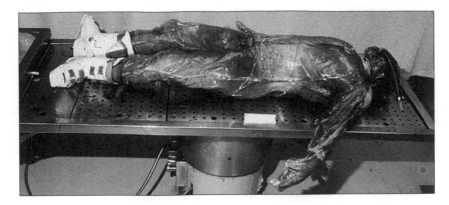

Figure 6.17 Under the winter garments, the body was wrapped from head to toe in a transparent homemade plastic jumpsuit sealed with duct tape. (From Sauvageau, A. and Racette, S. Courtesy of the editor, *J Forensic Sci* 2006;51(1):137–139.)

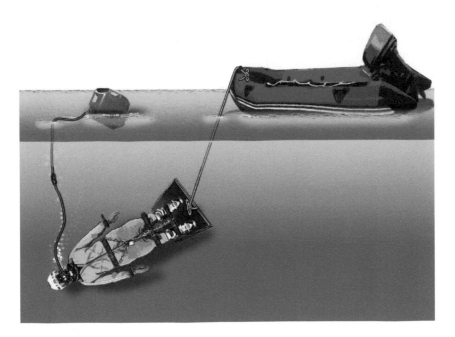

Figure 6.18 Aqua eroticum reconstruction. The wooden board was linked to a floating pneumatic boat by an electrical cord. The victim had linked a long black tube from his mouth to an open plastic container floating on the lake, thus creating a device for air supply. (Courtesy of the editor, *Journal of Forensic Science*, and courtesy of Medical Legal Art. Illustration copyright 2009 Medical Legal Art, http://www.doereport.com.)

Smothering

Smothering as a method of autoerotic asphyxia was reported only once. It seems that an autoerotic practitioner smothered himself with a pillow.[35] No further detail is available on this unusual case.

Case history: Smothering

A 66-year-old white male was discovered lying dead on his bed by police, who had been called to the man's apartment. The deceased was wearing women's clothing, which consisted of a gray turtleneck sweater with crotch snaps and red pantyhose (Figures 6.19a through 6.19e). The upper torso was bound with straps and chains, which were interconnected by a series of locks. A rubber mask covered his face, and the mask was connected to the bed board by rope. There was an electrical apparatus attached to a hook in the ceiling, which consisted of a timer and two wires. It was basically a homemade capacitor. This equipment was plugged into a wall socket. One of the wires extended to the crotch area of the victim. A copper wire loop had been fitted beneath the snaps of the turtleneck sweater and could be connected to the electrical device. In the man's room, police investigators discovered three suitcases full of women's undergarments, wigs, and "falsies," as well as other sexual paraphernalia consisting of dildos, discipline masks, and pornographic materials. When the body was examined, the victim was found to be wearing women's undergarments. Under the head mask, duct tape covered his eyes, foam rubber was stuffed in his mouth, and a headband held a small rubber ball in each ear. He was totally in the dark and could not hear a thing, but all of the bindings and chains were within his grasp. His escape mechanism was a single lock, which secured all of the chains wrapped around his body. The deceased had held the keys for this lock in his right hand. He had apparently dropped his keys on the floor, where the police discovered them. The duct tape and rubber balls in his ears certainly

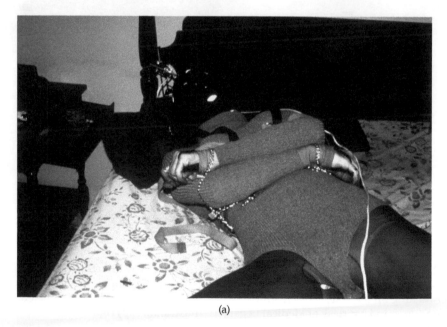

(a)

Figure 6.19 (a) Crime scene. This photo depicts a male dressed in female attire lying on a bed with a discipline mask over his head. (b) Victim in bondage. This photo shows the discipline mask and the bondage, consisting of ropes and chains. (c) Copper loop. This photo depicts the copper loop between the victim's legs, which was connected to the capacitor, which sent electrical charges to the copper wire. (d) Electrical capacitor. This photo shows the homemade capacitor attached to a socket in the ceiling, which sent the electrical charge to the copper wire. (e) Smothering. Autopsy photo depicts the duct tape and foam rubber on the victim's face. (Courtesy of Detective Lieutenant Raymond Krolak, Colonie, New York, Police Department, retired; from author Geberth's files.)

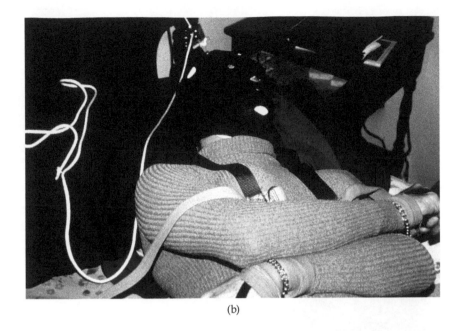

(b)

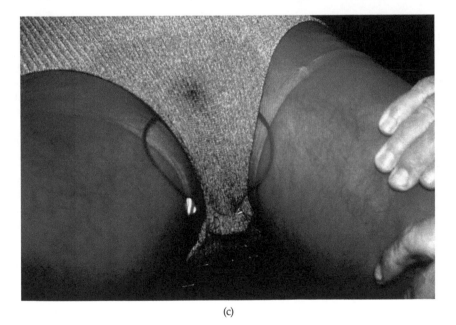

(c)

Figure 6.19 (continued) (a) Crime scene. This photo depicts a male dressed in female attire lying on a bed with a discipline mask over his head. (b) Victim in bondage. This photo shows the discipline mask and the bondage, consisting of ropes and chains. (c) Copper loop. This photo depicts the copper loop between the victim's legs, which was connected to the capacitor, which sent electrical charges to the copper wire. (d) Electrical capacitor. This photos show the home-made capacitor attached to a socket in the ceiling, which sent the electrical charge to the copper wire. (e) Smothering. Autopsy photo depicts the duct tape and foam rubber on the victim's face. (Courtesy of Detective Lieutenant Raymond Krolak, Colonie, New York, Police Department, retired; from author Geberth's files.)

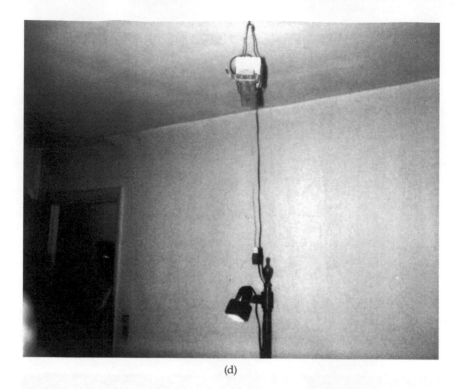

(d)

Figure 6.19 (continued) (a) Crime scene. This photo depicts a male dressed in female attire lying on a bed with a discipline mask over his head. (b) Victim in bondage. This photo shows the discipline mask and the bondage, consisting of ropes and chains. (c) Copper loop. This photo depicts the copper loop between the victim's legs, which was connected to the capacitor, which sent electrical charges to the copper wire. (d) Electrical capacitor. This photos show the home-made capacitor attached to a socket in the ceiling, which sent the electrical charge to the copper wire. (e) Smothering. Autopsy photo depicts the duct tape and foam rubber on the victim's face. (Courtesy of Detective Lieutenant Raymond Krolak, Colonie, New York, Police Department, retired; from author Geberth's files.)

shut out any possibility of seeing the keys or hearing them drop to the floor. He had been bound to the bed in such a manner that he would not have been able to reach the floor even if he had heard the keys drop. The cause of death was smothering. The police supervisor and the detective investigating this case had both been to one of the practical homicide investigation lectures of one of us. They immediately recognized the death to be an autoerotic fatality based on that information.

However, when the medical examiner of the jurisdiction arrived at the scene, he told the detectives it appeared to be a homicide related to "biker gang" activity. He obviously was not familiar with such cases and based his conclusion of homicide on the bizarre binding of the body. The medical examiner was shown additional references of these types of deaths from the practical homicide investigation textbook and ruled the death accidental.

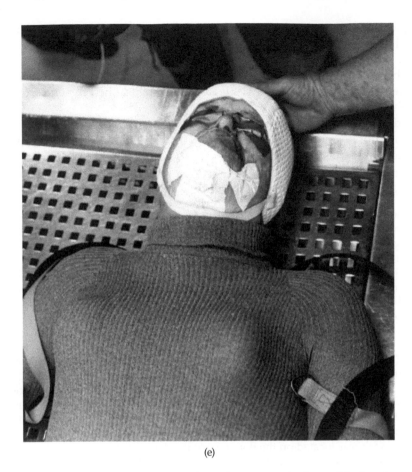

(e)

Figure 6.19 (continued) (a) Crime scene. This photo depicts a male dressed in female attire lying on a bed with a discipline mask over his head. (b) Victim in bondage. This photo shows the discipline mask and the bondage, consisting of ropes and chains. (c) Copper loop. This photo depicts the copper loop between the victim's legs, which was connected to the capacitor, which sent electrical charges to the copper wire. (d) Electrical capacitor. This photos show the home-made capacitor attached to a socket in the ceiling, which sent the electrical charge to the copper wire. (e) Smothering. Autopsy photo depicts the duct tape and foam rubber on the victim's face. (Courtesy of Detective Lieutenant Raymond Krolak, Colonie, New York, Police Department, retired; from author Geberth's files.)

Other atypical methods

Because sexual fantasies are quite diverse and to some extent unpredictable, it is impossible to establish a definitive list of atypical autoerotic methods. Forensic experts should therefore keep an open mind to recognizing creative, original, never-reported autoerotic methods. Before concluding the investigation of the autoerotic nature of such one-of-a-kind cases, a thorough investigation should be performed, with complete autopsy, toxicological analyses, complete scene investigation, and exhaustive police investigation.

Two examples of other atypical methods are found in the literature. Tan and Chao described the case of a 25-year-old man who was using the heat of a table lamp between his thighs to enhance his sexual pleasure.[36] The wire of the lamp had been stretched taut to allow it to reach the man, and an electrical problem ensued, causing death by electrocution. Even though the cause of death was autoerotic electrocution, the autoerotic method used for sexual pleasure enhancement was genital heat exposure. This form of sexual activity is generally innocuous and therefore is not frequently encountered in autoerotic deaths.

Another example was found in a study by Shields et al.[10] A 27-year-old man was found dead in his bed with a gunshot wound to the right side of the head. Evidence of masturbation before the gunshot led the investigators to conclude he engaged in an autoerotic practice of Russian roulette.

It should be remembered, however, that natural deaths occurring during autoerotic activity should not be considered autoerotic deaths. For example, death by an acute myocardial infarct while masturbating with a device does not constitute autoerotic death.

Case history: Positional asphyxia—washing machine

Police officers were summoned to a residence to check on the welfare of a 41-year-old man who had not reported to work for 2 days. There was no response at his house. Nothing was disturbed, and everything seemed fine. The television was on in the living room. All of the beds were made, and there was mail on the kitchen counter.

A check of the house proved negative, and everything seemed to be in place. The officers checked the basement and were getting ready to leave when they noticed a foot protruding from the top of a top-loading washing machine. Also visible was the buttocks portion of the body, which was wearing gray undershorts (Figures 6.20a and 6.20b).

The washing machine was a top-loading unit. It was still plugged in and powered up. The interior agitator components had been removed and were located on the floor nearby (Figure 6.21). The tools and removed bolts were found on an ironing board next to the dryer.

The body was head first into the washing tub and folded in a semifetal position. The victim's face, head, neck, and torso were not visible. Both legs were entirely inside the tub. Only the left foot protruded up and out of the tub. The deceased was clad in gray undershorts, a blue nylon sleeveless T-shirt, and one cotton sock on his right foot. The matching sock was located on the floor next to the dryer.

The body could not be removed from the tub. Crime scene officers had to dismantle the tub by cutting it apart using an electric Sawzall®, being careful not to touch the body (Figure 6.22). The outer fiberglass was removed first, and a hole was cut into the lower portion of the inner tub to drain out 24–30 quarts of water.

The inner tub was cut away in sections, avoiding blade contact with the body. Approximately half of the inner tub was removed, which allowed the body to be released and pulled out from the front. The body remained in a tucked/folded position when pulled free (Figure 6.23). Rigor mortis was almost absent, and the limbs could be straightened without much force.

The cloth materials in the bottom of the tub were two nonmatching bed sheets. The compression of the body could be seen in the sheets. The controls had been set for a wash cycle, medium load, warm wash/cold rinse.

Investigation revealed that the deceased had last been on his computer at 10:00 p.m. the previous evening and had logged off at 10:20 p.m. The position of the body inside the machine clearly indicated that the deceased had intentionally climbed head first into the tub and had gotten stuck in this situation. He had no way of extricating himself. The injuries and abrasions to his arms indicated that he had desperately struggled to free himself. Although the victim's head was down in the tub, the mouth and nose were not in the water, and drowning was not the cause of death. Seminal fluid was present in the victim's underwear.

The cause of death was positional asphyxia. The manner of death was ruled accidental. The autoerotic method used was atypical: creating a confinement of the body in a washing machine.

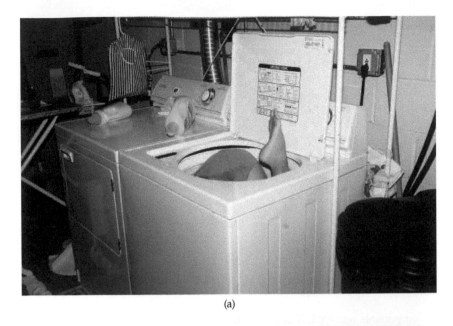

(a)

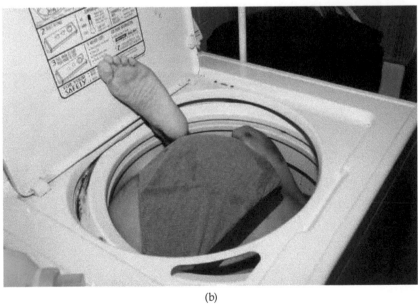

(b)

Figure 6.20 (a) and (b) Body in washing machine. The victim climbed into the tub of the machine headfirst. Only his left foot was protruding from the machine. (Courtesy of Detective Edward Davies, Montgomery Township, Pennsylvania, Police Department; from author Geberth's files.)

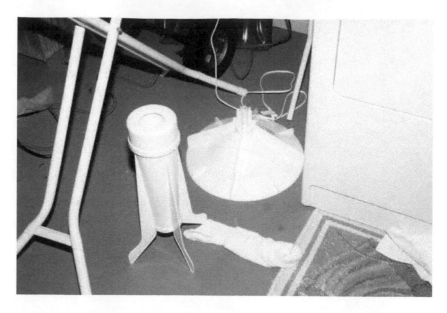

Figure 6.21 Components removed. Victim had removed the agitator and components to fit into the tub. (Courtesy of Detective Edward Davies, Montgomery Township, Pennsylvania, Police Department; from author Geberth's files.)

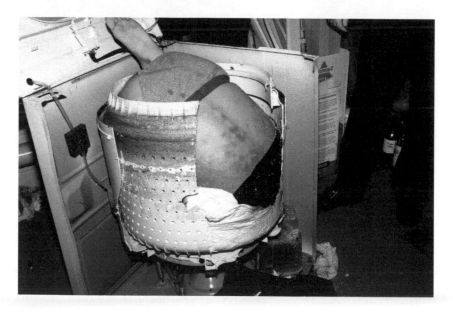

Figure 6.22 Body being removed. Police used a Sawzall® tool to remove the body intact. (Courtesy of Detective Edward Davies, Montgomery Township, Pennsylvania, Police Department; from author Geberth's files.)

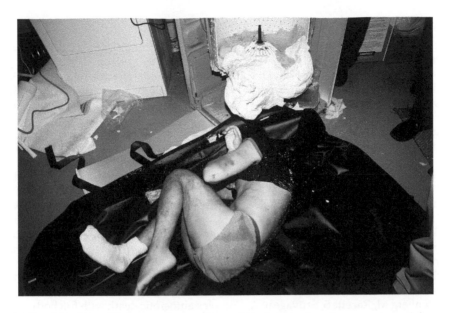

Figure 6.23 Fetal Position. This was the position of the body when it was removed from the tub. (Courtesy of Detective Edward Davies, Montgomery Township, Pennsylvania, Police Department; from author Geberth's files.)

Atypical methods of autoerotic deaths: Checklist for the forensic expert

- Keep in mind that autoerotic deaths are not restricted to hangings and plastic bags.
- Be aware that 5% to 10% of autoerotic deaths are atypical.
- List the atypical autoerotic methods as electrocution, overdressing/body wrapping, foreign body insertion, and atypical asphyxia methods.
- Know that, usually, autoerotic electrocutions are accidents involving self-made electric systems with low-voltage alternating current (domestic current) used to stimulate the nipples, the scrotum, the penis, or the anorectal region.
- Autoerotic electrocutions are usually related to a malfunction of the electrical device or to an accidental contact with a more active part of the circuit.
- Know that in overdressing/body wrapping, death can be caused by smothering or hyperthermia.
- Be aware that foreign body insertion is usually an innocuous practice, but in rare instances, immediate deaths by acute hemorrhage, obstruction of the airways, or air embolism have been reported or delayed deaths by an infectious process secondary to a trapped foreign body or to perforation of a hollow viscus.
- List atypical autoerotic asphyxia methods as ligature strangulation, chest compression, inverted or abdominal suspension, immersion and drowning, and smothering.
- Keep in mind that deaths from natural causes occurring during solitary sexual activity should not be classified as autoerotic deaths.

References

1. Sauvageau A, Racette S. Autoerotic deaths in the literature from 1954 to 2004: a review. *J Forensic Sci* 2006;51(1):140–146.
2. Sauvageau A. A revisitation of the most common methods of autoerotic activity leading to death based on the new standardized classification of asphyxia. *J Forensic Sci* 2011;56(1):261.
3. Sauvageau A. Autoerotic deaths: a 25-year retrospective epidemiological study. *Am J Forensic Med Pathol* 2012;33(2):143–146.
4. Wright RK. Death or injury caused by electrocution. *Clin Lab Med* 1983;3:343–353.
5. Klintschar M, Grabuschnigg P, Beham A. Death from electrocution during autoerotic practice: case report and review of the literature. *Am J Forensic Med Pathol* 1998;19(2):190–193.
6. Sivaloganathan S. Curiosum eroticum—a case of fatal electrocution during auto-erotic practice. *Med Sci Law* 1981;21(1):47–50.
7. Cairns FJ, Rainer SP. Death from electrocution during auto-erotic procedures. *N Z Med J* 1981;94(693):259–260.
8. Cooke CT, Cadden Ga, Margolius KA. 1994. Autoerotic deaths: four cases. *Pathology* 26:276–280.
9. Schott JC, Davis GJ, Hunsaker JC, 3rd. Accidental electrocution during autoeroticism. A shocking case. *Am J Forensic Med Pathol* 2003;24(1):92–95.
10. Shields LB, Hunsaker DM, Hunsaker JC, 3rd, Wetli CV, Hutchings KD, Holmes RM. Atypical autoerotic death: part II. *Am J Forensic Med Pathol* 2005;26(1):53–62.
11. Schellenberg M, Racette S, Sauvageau A. Complex autoerotic death with full body wrapping in a plastic body bag: a case report. *J Forensic Sci* 2007;52(4):954–956.
12. Johnstone JM, Hunt AC, Ward EM. 1960. Plastic-bag asphyxia in adults. *Br Med J* 1960;2(5214):1714–1715.
13. Mynyard F. Wrapped to death. Unusual autoerotic death. *Am J Forensic Med Pathol* 1985;6(2):151–152.
14. Eriksson A, Gezelius C, Bring G. Rolled up to death. An unusual autoerotic fatality. *Am J Forensic Med Pathol* 1987;8(3):263–265.
15. Madea B. Death in a head-down position. *Forensic Sci Int* 1993;61:119–132.
16. Byard RW, Eitzen DA, James R. Unusual fatal mechanisms in nonasphyxial autoerotic death. *Am J Forensic Med Pathol* 2000;21(1):65–68.
17. Sivaloganathan S. Catheteroticum. Fatal late complication following autoerotic practice. *Am J Forensic Med Pathol* 1985;6(4):340–342.
18. Marc B, Chadly A, Durigon M. Fatal air embolism during female autoerotic practice. *Int J Leg Med* 1990;104:59–61.
19. Sauvageau A, Boghossian E. Classification of asphyxia: the need for standardization. *J Forensic Sci* 2010;55(5):1259–1267.
20. Danto BL. A case of female autoerotic death. *Am J Forensic Med Pathol* 1980;1(2):117–121.
21. Byard RW, Hucker SJ, Hazelwood RR. Fatal and near-fatal autoerotic asphyxia episodes in women. Characteristics features based on a review of nine cases. *Am J Forensic Med Pathol* 1993;14(1):70–73.
22. Sauvageau A, Ambrosi C, Kelly S. Three non-lethal ligature strangulations filmed by an autoerotic practitioner: comparison of early agonal responses in strangulation by ligature, hanging and manual strangulation. *Am J Forensic Med Pathol* 2012;33(4):339–340.
23. Sauvageau A, LaHarpe R, King D, Dowling G, Andrews S, Kelly S, Ambrosi C, Guay JP, Geberth VJ. The Working Group on Human Asphyxia. Agonal sequences in fourteen filmed hangings with comments on the role of the type of suspension, ischemic habituation and ethanol intoxication on the timing of agonal responses. *Am J Forensic Med Pathol* 2011;32(2):104–107.
24. Sauvageau A, LaHarpe R, Geberth VJ. Agonal sequences in eight filmed hangings: analysis of respiratory and movement responses to asphyxia by hanging. *J Forensic Sci* 2010;55(5):1278–1281.
25. Sauvageau A, Ambrosi C, Kelly S. Autoerotic nonlethal filmed hangings: a case series and comments on the estimation of the time to irreversibility in hanging. *Am J Forensic Med Pathol* 2012;33(2):159–162.
26. Blanchard R, Hucker SJ. Age, transvestism, bondage, and concurrent paraphilic activities in 117 fatal cases of autoerotic asphyxia. *Br J Psychiatry* 1991;159:371–377.

27. Hazelwood RR, Burgess AW, Groth AN. Death during dangerous autoerotic practice. *Soc Sci Med* 1981;15E:129–133.
28. Sauvageau A, Desjarlais A, Racette S. Deaths in a head-down position: a case report and review of the literature. *Forensic Sci Med Pathol* 2008;4:51–54.
29. O'Halloran RL, Dietz PE. Autoerotic fatalities with power hydraulics. *J Forensic Sci* 1993;38(2):359–364.
30. Behrendt N, Modvig J. The lethal paraphiliac syndrome—accidental autoerotic death in Denmark 1933–1990. *Am J Forensic Med Pathol* 1995;16(3):232–237.
31. Thibault R, Spencer JD, Bishop JW, Hibler NS. An unusual autoerotic death: asphyxia with abdominal ligature. *J Forensic Sci* 1984;29(2):679–684.
32. Sivaloganathan S. Aqua-eroticum—a case of auto-erotic drowning. *Med Sci Law* 1984;24(4): 300–302.
33. Sauvageau A, Racette S. Aqua-eroticum: an unusual autoerotic fatality in a lake involving a home-made diving apparatus. *J Forensic Sci* 2006;51(1):137–139.
34. Breitmeier D, Mansouri F, Albrecht K, Böhm U, Tröger HD, Kleemann WJ. Accidental auto-erotic deaths between 1978 and 1997. Institute of Legal Medicine, Medical School Hannover. *Forensic Sci Int* 2003;137:41–44.
35. Diamond M, Innala SM, Ernulf KE. Asphyxiophilia and autoerotic death. *Hawaii Med J* 1990;49(1):11–16, 24.
36. Tan CT, Chao TC. A case of fatal electrocution during an unusual autoerotic practice. *Med Sci Law* 1983;23(2):92–95.

chapter seven

Atypical victims

Introduction

The typical victim of an autoerotic accident is a white adult male. In a 50-year review of the literature on autoerotic death, 96% of the victims were males, and 96% were white.[1] Female victims are rare, as are black, Asian, and Native victims. Most victims are adults, young to middle aged. Younger victims are not typical: Only 1% of the victims are less than 15 years of age, and the 15- to 19-year-old age group seems to represent only from 5% to 16% of the victims.[1,2] Elderly victims more than 65 years of age are also uncommon, with less than 1% of cases.[1,3]

In this chapter, we discuss four types of atypical victims: the female victim, the non-white victim, the teenage victim, and the elderly victim. A good understanding of these victims is essential for the forensic expert to avoid missing the autoerotic nature of these cases. It is our experience that without this understanding of the existence and particularities of atypical victims, investigators and medical examiners are misdirected toward assuming these cases must be suicidal or homicidal.

Female victims

Female victims are very rare, with fewer than 25 cases reported in the literature. It is probable that the actual number is higher since it is likely that cases are often missed because the presentation of the female victims is less obvious than the presentation of male ones. The scene in female victims is more subtle, usually without pornographic material, complex bindings, or cross-dressing. Accessory props are generally limited to foreign body insertion into the vagina or rectum.

Female victims in the early period of forensic literature on autoerotic deaths (1947 to 1980)

In the early period of the literature on autoerotic deaths (1947 to 1980; see Chapter 1), it was thought that female victims did not exist. In 1968, Camps stated that these cases "seem to occur exclusively in males."[4] In the early 1970s, Resnick wrote that this activity was reported only in males because it was due to some castration concerns.[5] Resnick wrote, "The absolute absence of females reinforces the theoretical position that this syndrome is related to phallic anxiety concerns. Females do engage in other behaviors that enhance sexual sensations but without neck specificity" (at that time, the notion of autoerotic deaths was still restricted to autoerotic hanging).

The first documented case of female autoerotic death seems to be the case reported by Henry in 1971 in the *Medico-Legal Bulletin*.[6] A 19-year-old girl had died of autoerotic strangulation caused by accidental malfunctioning of a part of her costume, resulting in unintentional strangulation. At the time, Henry wrote that female cases must be extremely rare as he was unable to find a single other report in the literature.

A few years later, in 1975, Sass reported a second case of female autoerotic death.[7] A 35-year-old divorcee was found by her daughter in the morning. The body was nude, hanging in a part-lying position; the body was lying on a shelf at the rear of a closet, with the torso, arms, and head hanging in the air in front of the shelf. A folded quilt was under her abdomen and upper thighs. An electric vibrator was between her legs at the vulva area. A clothespin was on the nipple of her right breast, and another clothespin was found immediately below her left breast.

A third case was reported in 1980 by Danto.[8] A 21-year-old black single woman was found dead, nude, on the floor of her bathroom in her secured apartment (the case was presented in further detail in Chapter 6). The body was kneeling at the bathtub, with the head underwater in the bath. Water had run out of the tub onto the bathroom floor. A sash cord was wrapped around her wrists, and another sash cord was wrapped several times around her neck. An iron bolt with a nut at the end was found under her buttocks. At autopsy, she was found to have died from aspiration of vomitus. An abrasion of the left forehead was also noticed. Danto presented his opinion that she had been masturbating with the iron bolt while creating asphyxia with the cord around her neck. She would have collapsed from the asphyxia and struck her head against the side of the bathtub, causing the forehead abrasion. She would have vomited from either the minor head trauma or the asphyxia, aspirated the gastric contents, and died.

Female victims in the golden age of forensic literature on autoerotic deaths (1981 to 1990)

In the article by Hazelwood et al.[9] that initiated the golden age of forensic literature on autoerotic deaths (see Chapter 1), the cases of three white females and one black female were mentioned as reviewed. However, there are no further details on these cases in the article. In their book of 1983, Hazelwood and his team[10] reported that they had reviewed 5 women's cases: 3 white women and 1 black woman between the ages of 20 and 29 and 1 white woman between the ages of 60 and 69. All these women died from autoerotic hanging, and none had presented any recognized paraphilia.

By the early golden age, the team of Hazelwood et al. started to envision what would later become the two main concepts of female autoerotic deaths: (1) These deaths do exist, although they are less common than for their male counterparts, and (2) the female autoerotic deaths are more subtle and do not usually present with the paraphilias so common in male autoerotic deaths.

In 1988, Byard and Bramwell[11] published a key article for the modern understanding of female autoerotic deaths. In this article, the authors reported that the usual props present at the scene of male cases, such as pornographic material, female undergarments, and elaborate bizarre equipment, might not be as common in female cases. Based on this more subtle presentation, they suggested that female cases might be underdiagnosed.

The comparative features of male and female autoerotic deaths were further explored in a following article by Byard et al. in 1990.[12] Their conclusions are presented in Table 7.1. Because women so rarely use pornography, complex bindings, and accessory props, the paucity of the scene renders the recognition of these cases as autoerotic more difficult, and there is a higher risk of confusion with homicide or suicide.

Table 7.1 Features of Male and Female Cases of Autoerotic Deaths

	Male	Female
Pornography	Yes	Rare
Unusual attire	Yes	Rare
Devices used to cause real or simulated pain	Yes	Rare
Bizarre props	Yes	No
Fetishisms	Yes	No

Source: Based on Byard RW, Hucker SJ, Hazelwood RR, *Forensic Sci Int* 1990;48(2):113–121.

Female victims in the modern era of forensic literature on autoerotic deaths (1991 to present)

After the publication of the two important articles by Byard et al.,[11,12] female cases continued to be reported from time to time.[13–18] From these cases, it seems that common female features are insertion of foreign bodies (in the vagina, rectum, or mouth) and the exposition of breast and genitals.

Currently, female cases of autoerotic death remain unusual, extremely challenging, and most probably largely unreported.

Case history: Typical autoerotic death—white female victim

The body of a 33-year-old white female, who had recently been laid off from work, was discovered in her locked apartment by an acquaintance, who became concerned when she could not make contact with her. The victim's friend, who had a key to the apartment, tried to get in but a dead bolt had been secured that could only be unlocked from inside. She then notified another friend, who requested the maintenance man of the building to assist in the entry. The maintenance man used a ladder to climb to the second floor balcony and entered the apartment through a sliding glass door. He then opened the apartment door from inside the apartment. The three individuals began to search the apartment and discovered the victim hanging from the top railing of the sliding glass shower door.

The victim was completely nude and was in a semistanding position. There was a restraint around the victim's torso that held her arms close to her body. The witnesses left the apartment and called 911 to report the death as a possible suicide. The first responders observed the woman hanging by the neck and determined that the victim had been dead for some time. Her body was cool to the touch, and livor mortis was present in her lower extremities. The responders properly did not cut her down or attempt any resuscitation, thereby preserving the death scene intact. The supervisor who noted that the victim's arms had been bound and her right wrist had a binding secured declared the death suspicious and designated the entire apartment a crime scene. All personnel were ordered out of the apartment, and investigators were notified in accordance with excellent practical homicide investigation procedure.

The reporting witnesses were interviewed. The victim's friend advised authorities that the victim had been laid off from work about a week earlier. The company had given her a generous severance package and was assisting her in finding employment. The victim was last seen by the reporting witness the previous evening and was in good spirits. The two of them had planned to go to a hockey game the next day. However, when the victim did not respond to several calls, the friend decided to check on her well-being and made the discovery.

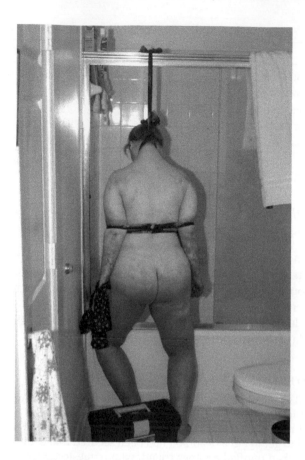

Figure 7.1 Female autoerotic. This close-up photograph shows the ligature around the victim's arms as well as the noose around her neck. The material hanging from her left wrist was probably used to secure her hands behind her back. (Courtesy of Instructor–Coordinator John J. Wiggins, North Carolina Criminal Justice Academy, Department of Justice, State of North Carolina. Reprinted with permission from V. J. Geberth, *Sex-Related Homicide and Death Investigation: Practical and Clinical Perspectives,* 2nd edition, CRC Press, Boca Raton, FL, 2010, p. 160.)

Investigators entered the apartment and examined the body. The victim was totally nude and hanging by the neck from the bathroom shower frame (Figure 7.1). The victim had a piece of cloth around her neck with a slipknot in it. The victim had another piece of cloth around her arms just above the elbows binding her arms to her side. There also was a piece of cloth tied around her left wrist. On the bathroom floor behind the victim was a set of black nipple clamps. On the floor in front of the victim was a large vibrator. On the bathroom sink, there was a vibrator dildo shaped like a penis (Figure 7.2). A search of the apartment revealed a number of sex toys and numerous items relating to sexual asphyxia, bondage, and autoerotic sexual activity (Figure 7.3). There were several pornographic magazines, bondage movies, and videos that were sexually graphic.

The medical examiner conferred with the investigators and agreed that the death was an autoerotic fatality. The examination of the victim's body did not reveal any assault or trauma, and the restraints used to bind the victim could easily be put on and removed by the victim herself. It was hypothesized that the victim had bound herself and used the ligature around her neck to restrict the oxygen flow to heighten the sensations she would receive while masturbating herself with the large vibrator found on the floor in front of her body. She most probably intended to stand up to relieve the pressure

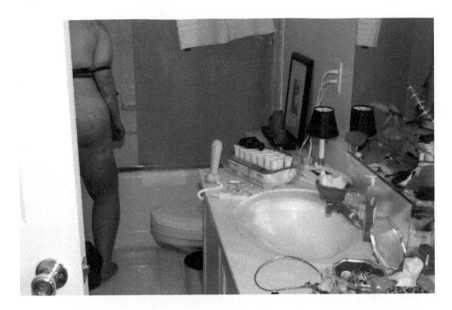

Figure 7.2 Paraphernalia: interior view of bathroom. A penis-shaped, battery-operated vibrator was on the bathroom sink vanity. (Courtesy of Instructor–Coordinator John J. Wiggins, North Carolina Criminal Justice Academy, Department of Justice, State of North Carolina. Reprinted with permission from V. J. Geberth, *Sex-Related Homicide and Death Investigation: Practical and Clinical Perspectives*, 2nd edition, CRC Press, Boca Raton, FL, 2010, p. 160.)

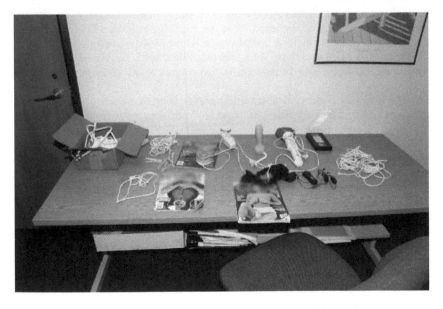

Figure 7.3 Sex toys. Various erotica and sex toys were recovered from the crime scene, such as vibrators, ropes, and nipple clamps. (Courtesy of John Wiggins, North Carolina Criminal Justice Academy, Department of Justice, State of North Carolina. Reprinted with permission from V. J. Geberth, *Sex-Related Homicide and Death Investigation: Practical and Clinical Perspectives*, 2nd edition, CRC Press, Boca Raton, FL, 2010, p. 161.)

on her neck from the noose but had misjudged the hypoxia, lost consciousness, and hung herself.

The case was properly classified as an autoerotic fatality and not a suicide as originally reported. The fact that the victim was discovered hanging nude in a bondage scenario, was heavily involved in solo sexual activity as evidenced by the number of sexual fantasy aids and sex toys recovered in the scene, coupled with the lack of any suicidal intent on the part of the victim made this case a classic sexual asphyxia event.

Case history: Female autoerotic death with acute cocaine toxicity

A 34-year-old woman was found dead in her secured apartment, kneeling and curled up behind the entrance door.[18] The door was locked from the inside, and there was no sign of break in. The body of the woman had to be pushed away from the locked door by the emergency staff trying to enter the apartment to check on her welfare.

The woman was dressed with a winter coat, leather jacket, sweater, and jeans but no underwear and no footwear. Her sweater was lifted over her head, exposing her breasts, and the jeans were unzipped. A syringe was found in the pocket of the coat, and another syringe was found on the floor near the body. A dog leash was wrapped loosely around her left arm and her neck. In the bathroom, multiple toothbrushes were found. This was unusual considering that the woman was living alone and presented a poor level of oral hygiene.

The woman was known for a past history of being abused as a youth. She was known for prostitution and drug use since her adolescence. She had then been abused by her previous spouse, and her children had been removed from her care by social services. She had a previous history of self-mutilation. She was HIV seropositive and on methadone treatment.

At the external examination, the body presented with moderate decomposition. The dog leash around the neck was loosely wrapped two times. The retractile mechanism of the leash was broken. A $20 bill was found stuffed in her mouth. A pair of scissors was inserted at the back of the jeans, near the right buttock. A $20 bill, a small piece of paper, and a small plastic bag containing a white powder were found at the vulva area, between the jeans and skin. A toothbrush soiled with feces had been inserted in the rectum by the brush end. In the vagina, a syringe, a small crumpled bag, and three syringe caps were found.

The autopsy did not reveal natural disease or trauma to account for the cause of death. A search for spermatozoids was negative. Toxicological analyses revealed cocaine toxicity.

That the cause of death was cocaine toxicity was rapidly agreed on by all the forensic team. The manner of death, however, was strongly argued, with supporters of homicide, suicide, and accidental overdose. None of these hypotheses could adequately explain all the elements from the scene. The presence of foreign body insertions and the double-looped dog leash around the neck would make no sense in a suicide or accidental overdose. If it had been a homicide, how could the aggressor leave the scene by locking the door from the inside, and how to explain the absence of violence on the body? A multidisciplinary team meeting was set up, and one of us was invited to review the case. The author presented a personal opinion that the case was in fact an autoerotic death. At the meeting, several senior police investigators admitted that they were unaware of the concept of female autoerotic death and thought the concept was restricted to males hanging themselves. The case was finally certified as accidental cocaine toxicity in the context of autoerotic death.

Non-white victims

A non-white victim is found in approximately 4% of cases.[1,3] In these atypical cases, the black race dominates, representing half of the non-white victims. Asians, Native Americans, and mixed races are less common. Apart from race, these cases do not seem to differ from the typical victims in any other aspect.

Teenager and elderly victims

The usual victim of autoerotic death is a male in his 30s. In a study reviewing all reported cases in the literature from 1954 to 2005, the average age of the male victim was 33 years (standard deviation of 15 years). Most victims are young to middle-aged adults. Younger victims are not typical: Only 1% of the victims are less than 15 years of age, and the group 15–19 years old seems to represent only from 5% to 16% of the victims.[1,2] The youngest autoerotic victim ever published was a young child, 9 years of age.[9] Elderly victims of more than 65 years of age are also uncommon, with less than 1% of cases.[1,3] The oldest autoerotic victim reported was an 89-year-old man.[19]

In teenage victims, the death investigation team is confronted with two important challenges. The first challenge is to avoid confusing autoerotic death and the nonsexual "choking game" activity. This term is unfortunately a misnomer,[20] and a better appellation would be strangulation game. The game is also known under a variety of slang names: fainting game, blackout, funky chicken, space monkey, cloud nine, black hole, passout, and others. In this dangerous game, children or adolescents use various ligatures (belts, shoelaces, dog collars) or their own hands or forearms to compress their own neck or the neck of a friend.

The strangulation game is usually not autoerotic in nature. The children play the game to test their fear, and there is no sexual content to their game. Sometimes, however, particularly in a compulsive solitary practitioner, it seems that the practice is more in line with an autoerotic asphyxiation than the typical strangulation game. In these cases, it is often difficult to determine if the accident is autoerotic in nature. This is particularly challenging considering that the death scene of a young autoerotic practitioner is usually poorer in forensic clues than the scene of the older practitioner, with on average only two scene features (see Chapter 3). Therefore, the presence of nudity or genital exposure at the scene of an apparent solitary strangulation game should be enough to at least raise the question about the possibility of an autoerotic event. However, this will not change the cause and manner of death, as they will remain the same in both the strangulation game and the autoerotic death: strangulation as the cause of death (ligature strangulation in most cases) and accident as the manner of death.

Victims of autoerotic activity who are more than 65 years of age are extremely rare, with fewer than 10 cases in the forensic literature (9,15,19,20–24). Because of their rarity, little is known about theses cases. It is probably that they do not differ significantly from the more classical cases apart from the age of their victims.

Case history: Equivocal death—black female victim

One of us was involved with an equivocal death investigation involving the hanging death of a 17-year-old black female. A detective was concerned that the medical examiner and other detectives had classified this case as a suicide. He felt, based on his investigation into the background of the victim and what he observed at the scene, that the death might have been an autoerotic fatality. The detective was concerned that the family was blaming themselves for the daughter's death. One of us reviewed his case file and crime scene photos and provided the detective with a full report, which he provided to his superiors and the medical examiner for review.

The location of the incident was in the basement of a single-family home occupied by the deceased and her family. The victim was home alone at the time of the incident. The area that the victim selected was secluded from the rest of the home. There was no evidence of any break-in or entry. The victim, who was found by her brother, had been hanging from a wire noose, which had been affixed to a rusty metal clothes rod. There was a white towel wrapped around the victim's neck, which would have formed padding between the wire and her neck (Figure 7.4a). The victim was nude from the waist up and was wearing a pair of black sweatpants. A white T-shirt was observed approximately 6 feet away and appeared to have been discarded by the deceased. A white 5-gallon bucket was observed lying on its side near the area where the deceased was found (Figure 7.4b). Forensic examination of this bucket revealed latent prints, which were later identified as belonging to the right foot of the deceased. The material on the deceased's hands turned out to be rust from the metal pipe to which the wire had been affixed.

The deceased was a healthy and apparently happy 17-year-old young woman. The investigation disclosed that the deceased came from a family background in which both the mother and the stepfather provided parental guidance and support. The family consisted of the 17-year-old victim, her 19-year-old brother, the victim's mother, and her stepfather. In addition, the inquiry into the victim's background indicated that the victim maintained good social relationships with peers and was performing well in school.

The interview of the deceased's best friend indicated that the victim was popular and well liked. The victim had two boyfriends and was sexually promiscuous with another young man. There was no indication in the reports that the deceased was depressed or suicidal. Investigative considerations were the following: A teenage female victim was found partially nude in a secluded area of the house when no one was home. The location that the victim selected afforded her an opportunity to engage in a private fantasy. The most common method practiced in sexual asphyxia is hanging. There was some sort of padding between the neck and ligature to prevent any markings. This suspension point was within the reach of the deceased (rust on hands) until the plastic bucket was knocked over. It is a known fact that most victims of suicide are not found partially or fully nude. In this case, the victim's breasts were exposed.

The detective took this report and conferred with his superiors and the medical examiner. Reportedly, the medical examiner's initial concern about classifying this case as accidental was that the deceased did not fit the stereotypical profile of a practitioner of autoeroticism because she was a black female. However, the professional in-depth investigation undertaken by the detective provided enough factual basis to have this case reclassified. The consultative report simply validated the detective's hypothesis. The important point here is that the detective's dedication to properly classify this case as accidental provided a measure of consolation to the surviving family. The family was advised that the daughter did not commit suicide. The cause of death was hanging. The medical examiner reclassified the death from suicide to undetermined.

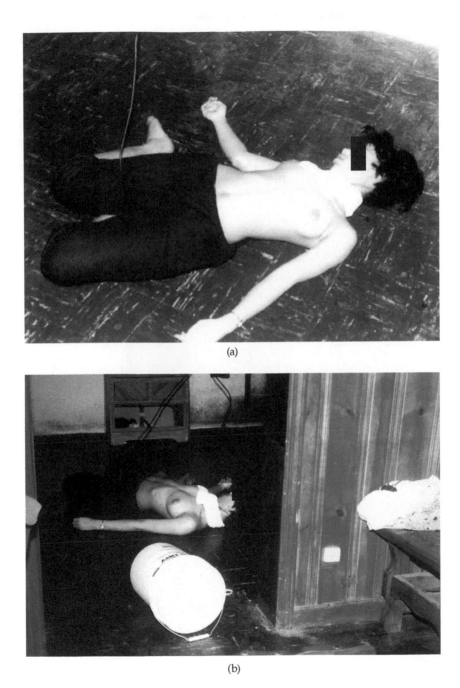

(a)

(b)

Figure 7.4 (a) Crime scene. The victim, reported as a victim of a suicide, was actually an autoerotic fatality. She was found hanging from an electrical wire that had been fastened into a noose. The victim was nude from the waist up and had placed padding between her neck and the noose to prevent any markings. (b) Plastic bucket. She had been standing on a plastic bucket as she engaged in this autoerotic activity, and the bucket had apparently slipped out from under her feet. (Courtesy of Detective Steven Little, Columbus, Ohio, Police Department; submitted from author Geberth's files.)

Case history: Autoerotic death—87-year-old male

This case involved an 87-year-old white male who was discovered after police went to his home on a request by the man's employer to check on his welfare. The victim had failed to show for work, and according to the employer, the victim was like an ox and had never missed a day of work.

The police officers attempted to make contact with the resident by knocking on the doors and windows of the house but did not get any response. The officers also attempted to call, but there was no answer. A decision was made to force entry, and the officers entered the kitchen as they called the resident's name. As the officers entered the living room area, they saw the man.

The victim was completely naked and bound in a standing position from his lower legs to the midchest with three different ropes (Figures 7.5 and 7.6). The ropes on the

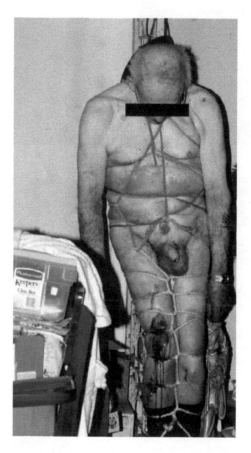

Figure 7.5 Elderly male. This 87-year-old male was discovered after police were called to "check on his welfare." The victim was completely naked and bound in a standing position from his lower legs to the midchest with three different ropes. The ropes on the man's legs were looped around each other from the feet up to the chest, creating a crisscross pattern. There was a belt around the rope behind the man's head, and a second belt was at the victim's feet. Detectives discovered a suitcase in the victim's bedroom closet, which contained ropes and belts similar to the ones on the victim, suggesting prior autoerotic activity on the part of the deceased. (Courtesy of Detective Ronald Antonucci, Wayne Township, New Jersey, Police Department. Reprinted with permission from V. J. Geberth, *Sex-Related Homicide and Death Investigation: Practical and Clinical Perspectives*, 2nd edition, CRC Press, Boca Raton, FL, 2010, p. 124.)

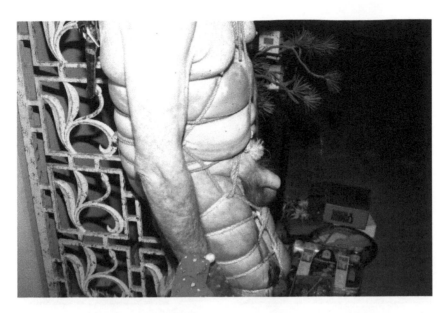

Figure 7.6 Bindings. A fourth rope was tied to the same wrought iron room divider and was around the neck of the victim. The rope around the victim's neck was loose but tightened when the victim's head was in a forward position. The victim's hands and genitals were free from the bindings. The ropes and bindings suggested that the victim was able to achieve this without assistance and had done this many times before. (Courtesy of Detective Ronald Antonucci, Wayne Township, New Jersey, Police Department. Reprinted with permission from V. J. Geberth, *Sex-Related Homicide and Death Investigation: Practical and Clinical Perspectives,* 2nd edition, CRC Press, Boca Raton, FL, 2010, p. 125.)

man's legs were looped around each other from the feet up to the chest, creating a criss-cross pattern. Two of the ropes were looped through and connected to a wrought iron room divider in the living room. These ropes held the man in a standing position. A fourth rope was tied to the same wrought iron room divider and was around the neck of the victim.

The victim's hands and genitals were free from the bindings. There was a belt around the rope behind the man's head, and a second belt was at the victim's feet. The rope around the victim's neck was loose but tightened when the victim's head was in a forward position. The victim could increase or release pressure by moving his head up and down.

The victim had apparently tied the first yellow rope around his ankles and then connected a second rope up his legs by looping each wrap as the ropes ascended to the waist. The rope was also looped through the wrought iron room divider and supported the victim's body. The third rope was connected to this series of ropes through the wrought iron divider up to the victim's midchest and then looped around his neck. The ropes and bindings suggested that the victim was able to achieve this without assistance and had done this many times before.

The detectives also discovered a suitcase in the victim's bedroom closet that contained ropes and belts similar to the ones on the victim, suggesting prior autoerotic activity on the part of the deceased (Figure 7.7).

The crime scene investigators used alternate lighting and discovered evidence of sexual activity. Semen was found on the floor in front of the victim as well as on the fingers of his right hand. Detectives and crime scene personnel examined the home, which was cluttered with boxes, old furniture, and various items and collectibles. There was no evidence of foul play or any criminal activity. The only damage or evidence of entry

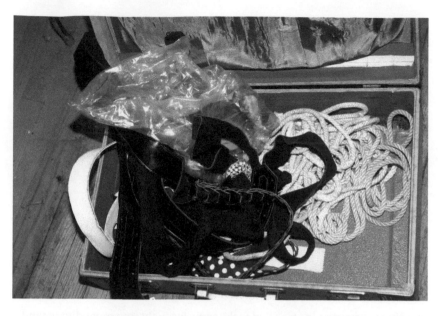

Figure 7.7 Paraphernalia. Detective discovered a suitcase in the victim's bedroom containing auto-erotic paraphernalia consisting of ropes and belts similar to the ones on the victim, suggesting prior autoerotic activity. (Courtesy of Detective Ronald Antonucci, Wayne Township, New Jersey, Police Department; submitted from author Geberth's files.)

into the home was through the door, which had been forced open by the police officers who originally responded to the call.

Investigation at the scene and subsequent medical examination revealed this case was an accidental death due to autoerotic activity. The unusual aspect of this case was the advanced age of the victim.

Case history: Autoerotic death—black female victim originally reported as a suicide

Police officers responded to a report of a "suicide" at a residence, which was a three-story townhouse in a middle- to upper-class neighborhood. The victim was a 17-year-old black female who was found hanging by her neck from a ligature tied to the bunk bed in her bedroom. The victim had a young sister, who had her own bedroom. The mother was employed, and the stepfather was a football coach. The family was actively involved in their church.

The stepfather had discovered his daughter hanging from the bunk bed and had managed to undo the ligature and place the girl's body on the floor, where he performed CPR. He called 911 for assistance, and the fire department had to make forcible entry since the man was attempting CPR in the upstairs bedroom. She was pronounced dead at the scene by paramedics.

Detectives were called to the scene to investigate this unattended death and were advised by the patrol sergeant that the case was a suicide. The blinds in the room were closed, and the lights were off. There was still light in the room, but with the blinds closed, there was not much light.

Detectives noted that the room was neat and clean, and that the bed was a bunk bed with the underneath part a desk area. The desk area had college information on it, and the computer was open to a social network page. The investigators scrolled down the social network page and noted that there were no recent entries or blogs indicating suicide or ending life. There was no suicide note.

The stepfather was interviewed; he advised that he noticed his stepdaughter's car was still in the garage, and it was past the time she would usually have left for work. He went upstairs, but the bedroom door was locked. He knocked but received no answer. He was able to pry the door open and entered the room. He advised the detectives that he saw the covers were bundled up on the top bunk and figured she was sleeping. He reached up there to shake her, but she was not in the bed. As he turned to his left, he noticed that she was hanging from the side of the bed. He undid a scarf that was around her neck and placed her on the floor in an attempt to start CPR. At first, he did not notice her hanging from the side of the bed because the blinds were closed, and no lights were on in the room. He had last seen her doing laundry after she worked on a school project approximately an hour earlier. The mother had last spoken to her daughter by phone at about the same time, and the girl told her mother she was doing some laundry.

The female's body was on the floor and had been covered with a sheet by the ambulance crew. The detectives removed the sheet and observed the deceased, who had an airway device still attached to her mouth along with two electrodes attached to her body, placed by the paramedics, who had attempted emergency resuscitation (Figure 7.8). The victim was wearing a black T-shirt with white lettering, "Blue Pride,"

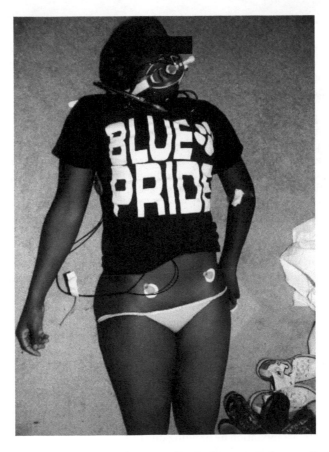

Figure 7.8 Body in crime scene. Police and paramedics had responded to a call of a possible suicide. The victim was pronounced dead, and detectives were asked to respond and conduct a basic death investigation. The victim was 17 years old and was discovered hanging by a scarf from her bunk bed. (Courtesy of Detective Mark Quagliarello, Homicide Unit, Raleigh, North Carolina, Police Department; submitted from author Geberth's files.)

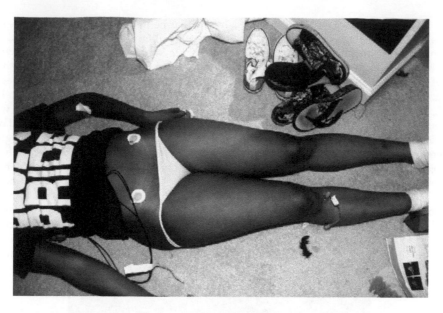

Figure 7.9 Body in crime scene. Detectives took into consideration the attire of the victim and the fact that she had been in her locked room hanging from a scarf and the fact that the victim had no history of depression. (Courtesy of Detective Mark Quagliarello, Homicide Unit, Raleigh, North Carolina, Police Department; submitted from author Geberth's files.)

and light blue panties (Figure 7.9). The ligature was a scarf, which was lying on a chair in the bedroom (Figure 7.10).

After the processing unit finished with initial photographs, the lead investigator did a formal search and inspection of the room and noticed that on the other side of the bed the sheet was tied around the metal railing (Figure 7.11). This seemed odd, and at first the detective thought that the sheet was tied around the railing possibly because of a prior suicide attempt.

The detective then noticed an object protruding from the vaginal area of the decedent when the body was placed into body bag. On closer examination, it was revealed to be a vibrator (Figure 7.12).

The initial inspection of the body indicated no signs of trauma. However, with the discovery of the vibrator and the ligatures tied to the bed, the lead investigator believed that this death may not have been a suicide but an accidental death.

The victim's computer was seized for further investigation. The results of the search warrant for the computer revealed Google searches for "choking game," "choking fetish," and "erotic asphyxiation" dating as far back as approximately a year. The hard drive of the computer indicated over 100 hits for these items. Numerous porn sites were located that were related to the fetish lifestyle. Several entries from a Yahoo chat line were also noted. Entries indicated she went by the screen name "Black-Crusade," and in a prior chat she had noted to someone that she "realized she had erotic asphyxiation fetish," and the subject responded, "I know you do."

The autopsy revealed no signs of sexual assault, and the cause of death was listed as consistent with asphyxiation by hanging due to autoerotic asphyxiation. The medical examiner ruled the death accidental.

The family was advised of the investigative and medical examiner's findings. Although they were still upset by the death of their daughter, they indicated that it would ease their suffering and make them sleep better knowing their daughter did not kill herself.

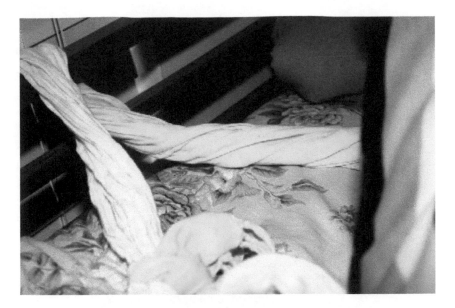

Figure 7.10 The ligature. This scarf was the ligature that the victim was using during her autoerotic activities. This scarf was taken as evidence. (Courtesy of Detective Mark Quagliarello, Homicide Unit, Raleigh, North Carolina, Police Department; submitted from author Geberth's files.)

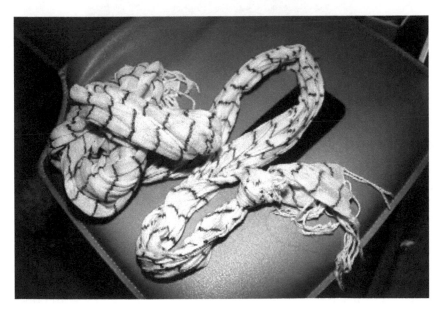

Figure 7.11 An additional ligature. Detective also noticed an additional ligature secured to the victim's bed, which further raised suspicions that the death might not have been a suicide. (Courtesy of Detective Mark Quagliarello, Homicide Unit, Raleigh, North Carolina, Police Department; submitted from author Geberth's files.)

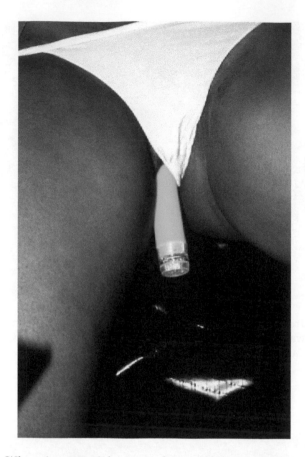

Figure 7.12 Vibrator. When the victim's body was being lifted onto the gurney, detectives noticed a green vibrator protruding through the victim's underwear. The discovery of this vibrator coupled with the other evidence at the scene led the investigators to suspect that the death was accidental. (Courtesy of Detective Mark Quagliarello, Homicide Unit, Raleigh, North Carolina, Police Department; submitted from author Geberth's files.)

Atypical victims: Checklist for the forensic expert

- Be aware that four types of atypical victims can be encountered: female victims, non-white victims, teenage victims, and elderly victims
- Be aware that while the deaths of non-white victims and elderly victims probably present similar scenes to the typical victims, the scenes in female victims and teenage victims are not as rich with forensic clues and easier to misinterpret.
- In female victims, the scene is more subtle, usually without pornographic material, complex bindings, and cross-dressing. Accessory props are generally limited to foreign body insertion into the vagina or rectum.
- In teenage victims, the scene usually has fewer forensic clues, with only two scene features on average.

References

1. Sauvageau A, Racette S. Autoerotic deaths in the literature from 1954 to 2004: a review. *J Forensic Sci* 2006; 51(1):140–146.
2. Sauvageau A. Autoerotic deaths: a 25-year retrospective epidemiological study. *Am J Forensic Med Pathol* 2012;33(2):143–146.
3. Sauvageau A, Geberth VJ. 2009. Elderly victim: an unusual autoerotic fatality involving an 87-year-old male. *Forensic Sci Med Pathol* 2009;5(3):233–235.
4. Brittain R. In Camps, FE (ed.), *Gradwohl's Legal Medicine*. Bristol, UK: Wright, 1968, Chapter 25, p. 549–552.
5. Resnick HLO. Erotized repetitive hangings: a form of self-destructive behaviour. *Am J Psychotherapy* 1972;26(1):4–21.
6. Henry RD. *Medico-Legal Bulletin*. Office of the Chief Medical Examiner, Department of Health, State of Virginia, 1971; Bulletin 214, 20(2).
7. Sass FA. Sexual asphyxia in the female. *J Forensic Sci* 1975; 20(1):181–185.
8. Danto BL. A case of female autoerotic death. *Am J Forensic Med Pathol* 1980:1:117–121.
9. Hazelwood RR, Burgess AW, Groth AN. Death during dangerous autoerotic practice. *Soc Sci Med* 1981;15E:129–133.
10. Hazelwood RR, Dietz PE, Burgess AW (eds.). *Autoerotic Fatalities*. Lexington, MA: Lexington Books, Heath, 1983.
11. Byard RW, Bramwell NH. Autoerotic death in females—an underdiagnosed syndrome? *Am J Forensic Med Pathol* 1988;9:252–254.
12. Byard RW, Hucker SJ, Hazelwood RR. A comparison of typical death scene features in cases of fatal male and female autoerotic asphyxia with a review of the literature. *Forensic Sci Int* 1990;48(2):113–21.
13. Marc B, Chadly A, Durigon M. Fatal air embolism during female autoerotic practice. *Int J Leg Med* 1990;104:59–61.
14. Byard RW, Hucker SJ, Hazelwood RR. Fatal and near-fatal autoerotic asphyxial episodes in women. *Am J Forensic Med Pathol* 1993;14(1):70–73.
15. Behrendt N, Modvig J. The lethal paraphiliac syndrome—accidental autoerotic death in Denmark 1933–1990. *Am J Forensic Med Pathol* 1995;16(3):232–237.
16. Gosink PD, Jumbelic MI. Autoerotic asphyxiation in a female. *Am J Forensic Med Pathol* 2000;20(3):114–118.
17. Shields LB, Hunsaker DM, Hunsaker JC, 3rd, Wetli CV, Hutchins KD, Holmes RM. Atypical autoerotic death: part II. *Am J Forensic Med Pathol* 2005;26(1):53–62.
18. Sauvageau A, Racette S. Female autoerotic deaths—still often overlooked: a case report. *Med Sci Law* 2006;46(4):357–359.
19. Müller K, Ottens R, Püschel K. [Death of an 89-year-old man during autosexual activity]. *Arch Kriminol* 2011;228(5–6):171–176.
20. Sauvageau A. The choking game: a misnomer. *Pediatr Emerg Care* 2010;26(12):965.
21. Walsh FM, Stahl CJ, III, Unger HT, Lilienstern OC, Stephens RG II. Autoerotic asphyxial deaths: a medicolegal analysis of forty-three cases. *Leg Med Annu* 1977;155–182.
22. Breitmeier D, Mansouri F, Albrecht K, Böhm U, Tröger HD, Kleemann WJ. Accidental autoerotic deaths between 1978 and 1997. Institute of Legal Medicine, Medical School Hannover. *Forensic Sci Int* 2003;137:41–44.
23. Cooke CT, Cadden GA, Margolius KA. Autoerotic asphyxiation: four cases. *Pathology* 1994;26:276–280.
24. Sauvageau A, Geberth VJ. Elderly victim: an unusual autoerotic fatality involving an 87-year-old male. *Forensic Sci Med Pathol* 2009; 5(3):233–235.

Index